AF229725

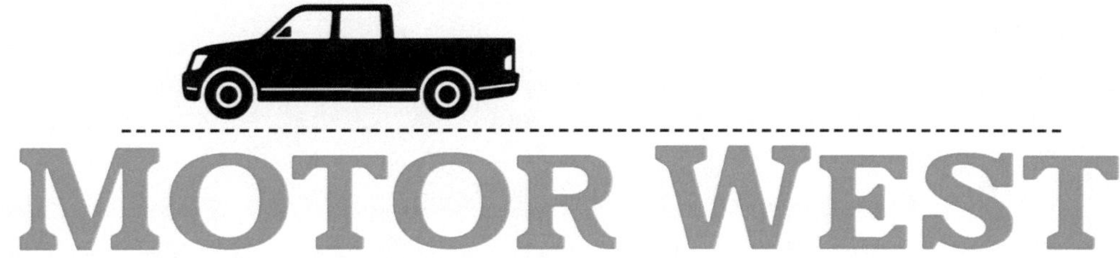

MOTOR WEST

A Route 66 Ramble Across America

Text and Photographs by
Barbara Brannon & Kay Ellington

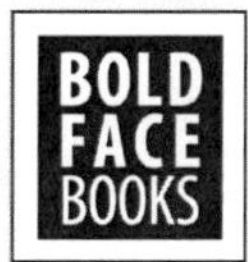

Spur, Texas • 2026

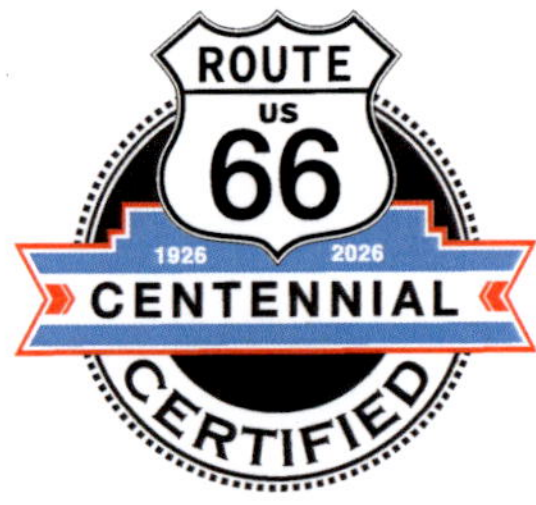

Motor West: A Route 66 Ramble Across America
Text copyright © 2026 by Barbara Brannon and Kay Ellington
Photographs copyright © 2026 by Barbara Brannon or Kay Ellington, except where otherwise indicated

Boldface Books, April 2026
An imprint of Winoca Books & Media
P. O. Box 430, Spur, Texas, 79370-0430
Printed in the United States of America

ISBN 978-1-935619-66-6
1 2 3 4 5   30 29 28 27 26

This book was set in the Abril and Methia West display faces and Minion and Myriad body faces in Adobe InDesign for the Macintosh computer. Cover and interior design were produced by The Paragraph Ranch.

Reach out to us at Route66Ramble@gmail.com
View more photos and related rambles at www.Route66Ramble.com

ON THE COVER Route 66 map, U.S. National Parks Service; individual photographs drawn from interior of this book.

For all the Roadies
with gratitude

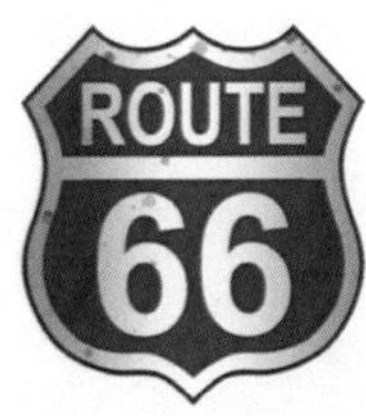

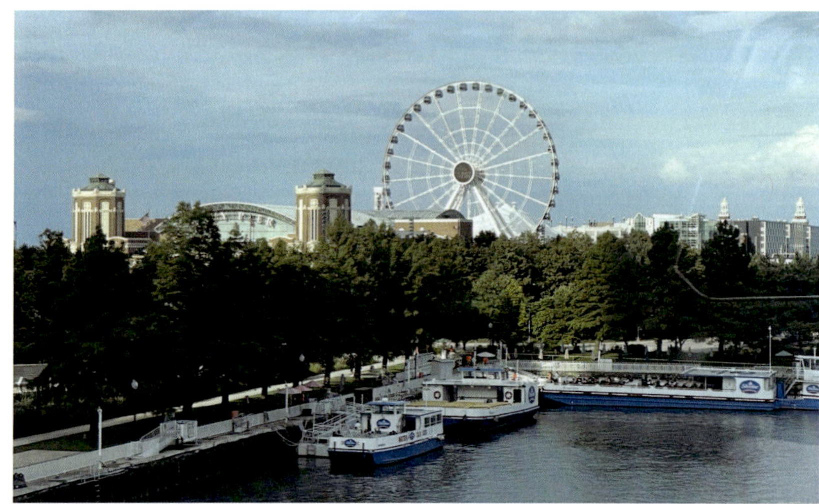

PIER TO PIER From the shore of Lake Michigan within view of the Navy Pier's famous Ferris wheel in Chicago 2,448 miles (give or take a few) across the U.S. to within a stone's throw of the Santa Monica Pier west of Los Angeles, Route 66 rewards the intrepid traveler with sights and insights.

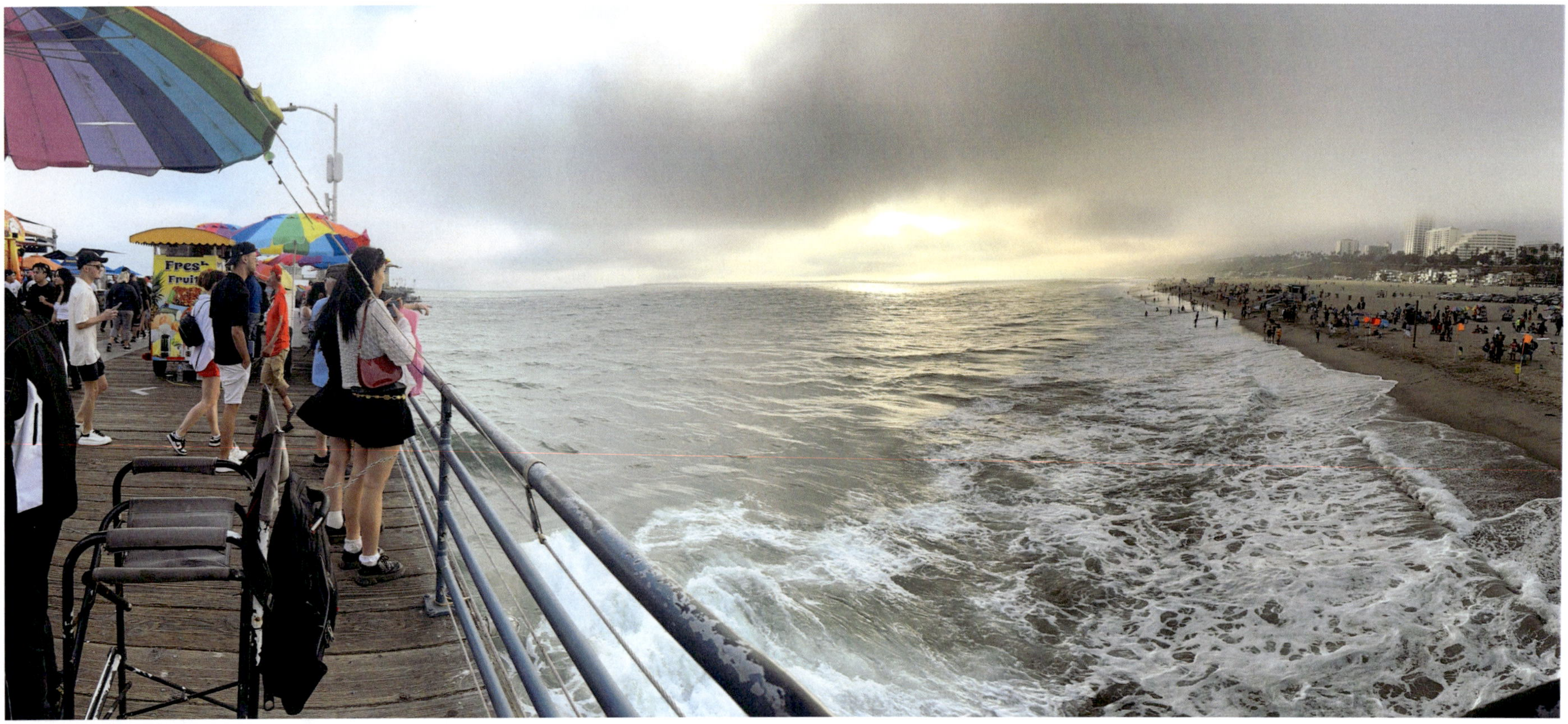

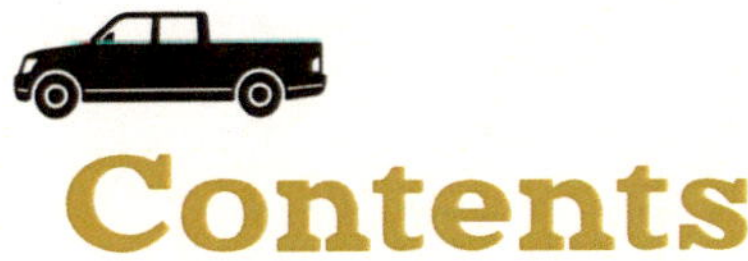

Contents

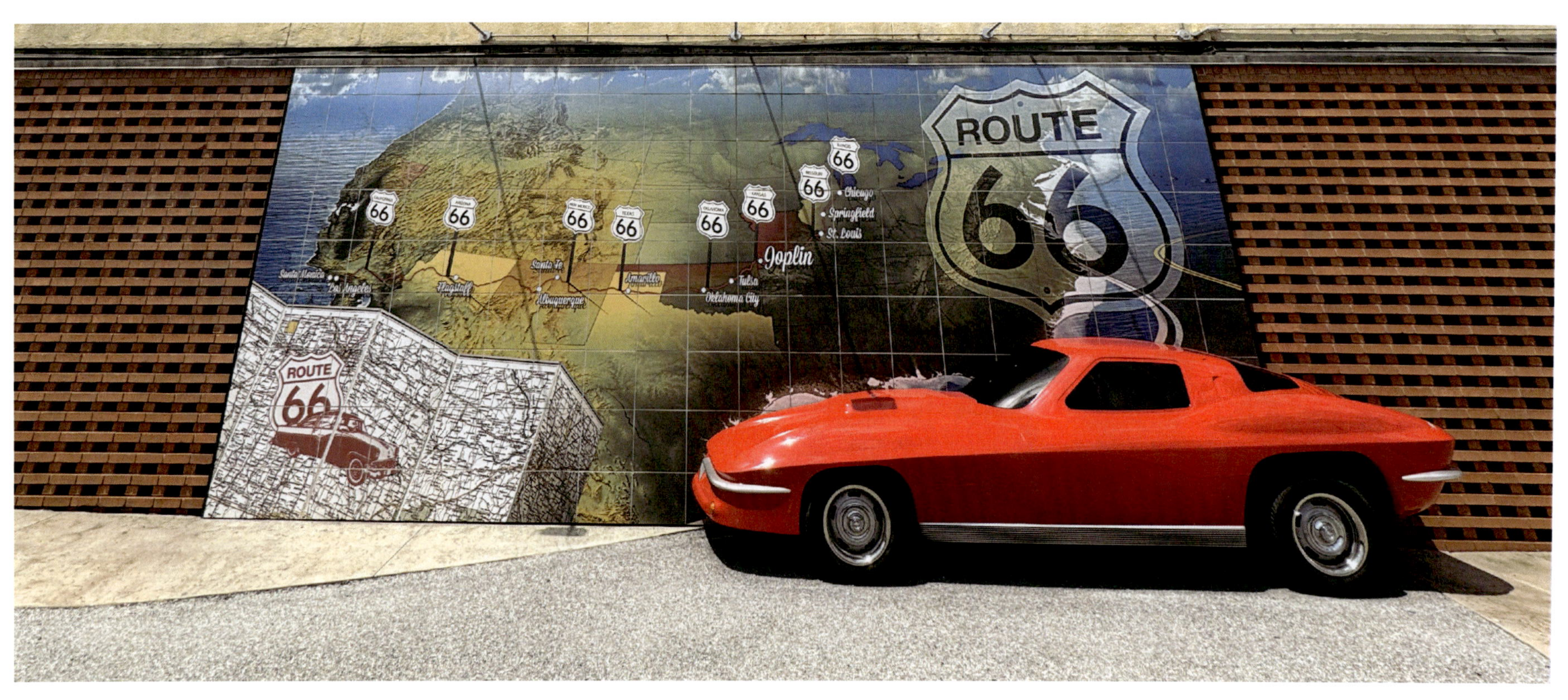

ROUTE 66 IN 3-D Yes, the sports car (only half of one, actually) is part of the art installation on the Pearl Bros. building in Joplin, Missouri.

Roads go ever ever on

I'M A WANDERER BY NATURE. Perhaps it's my inheritance, as the eldest child in a middle-class American family that had the freedom to take discretionary road trips in an era when the discretionary road trip was what middle-class families did. Perhaps the wanderlust was born from the adventures of reading—on rainy days when the library provided a virtual universe to explore and on sunny ones that provided actual roads to ride on two wheels. I remember afternoons turning the pages of entries and maps in the *Compton's Encyclopedia* volume by alphabetical volume in the babysitter's home just as eagerly as I might hop on my bicycle and follow the next unknown suburban street or country lane—simply to see where it went.

But travel eventually became a more intentional undertaking, one abetted by the benefit of salary and professional allowance. Going to a new place, or revisiting a familiar one, yielded the opportunity for deeper contemplation. Whatever the nominal purpose of a trip, the underlying goal was *discovery.*

Such discovery didn't have to be pioneering; after all, by the mid–twentieth century few places on Earth remained unexplored, and humanity was on the verge of venturing past the planet's atmosphere as well. It needed be new only to each new seeker.

I was well along in my travel life before I discovered Route 66 and its devotees, the Roadies. As a native Southerner, I hadn't yet had cause to explore that part of America's story.

When I came to Texas, all that changed. Locals called the region of the Lone Star State in which I'd landed the Panhandle, a concept I couldn't quite grasp. Florida and Oklahoma possessed extensions one could reach out and grab, maybe flip a hoecake with. But the shape of Texas did not evoke that analogy in my mind. Once it was laid out to me that the squared-off chimney at the top was the feature that gave this flattened, featureless geography its nickname, I had to drive it and see for myself.

That a canyon as ragged and wide as the Palo Duro might gouge through the heart of this country astonished me as well. And likewise did the revelation that a storied two-lane blacktop skirted its fringes, cutting a swath clear across that inscrutable Panhandle, half its mileage from the Great Lakes completed and the other half to the Pacific Ocean remaining over the western horizon.

I was hooked.

My new post with the Texas Historical Commission gave me the canyon as an office and those 178 miles of the Mother Road as a commute. Thus, in the year that representatives of the Road Ahead Partnership visited Amarillo to spread the eschatology of a rapidly approaching

> *Whatever the nominal purpose of a trip, the underlying goal was* discovery. *Such discovery didn't have to be pioneering … it needed be new only to each new seeker.*

Route 66 Centennial, I heeded the missionary call. I joined up. I became a disciple of road heritage, a student of linear resources, an advocate for federal preservation funding, state designations, wayfinding signage, original pavement, oral histories, and contributing structures. Yet I still hadn't driven the Route for myself, not all of it.

My familiarity had been limited to a 2003 road-trip assignment with a (then) *New York Times* regional newspaper in Wilmington, North Carolina, to chronicle what the completion of Interstate 40 had done for—or to—the cross-country experience that began right outside the gates of the university where I taught. Even on that most determined of anti–Route 66 journeys, once I reached Oklahoma City I was inexorably drawn to stretches of Mother Road pavement that were just too good to pass up.

And then, some years after I'd departed the enviably situated coastal Carolina city for the arid Texas plain and the promotion of the Panhandle became my paying job, I visited Route 66 towns often from Shamrock to Glenrio. I still lacked the perspective of the Chicago-to-LA through-drive, though, and I could only envision it in my imagination as a discrete set of waypoints in the Bobby Troup song.

So in 2024, after I'd returned to the week-in, week-out life of writing and editing and a stretch of flex-time opened up in my summer schedule, there was never any doubt in my mind what I wanted to do during my 66th trip around the sun.

My partner and I, by then co-publishers of a group of small weekly newspapers in Texas, had become adept at working from the road. We had a reliable team capable of staying on top of things back home, and for that we thank them sincerely.

We'd banked hotel points all year and freed up the credit cards. We'd repaired the extended-cab Ford pickup after the hail damage suffered in Colorado on her last road trip. We'd arranged for extended cat-sitting, and for that we sincerely thank our surrogate pet parents.

In keeping with the tradition of that 2003 *Wilmington Star-News* series, I planned to file stories about our experience from the road. Unlike the high-pressure situation of writing for a daily, though, Kay and I had the relative leisure of running one story per week in our series, from summer well into autumn.

We crafted a separate journey of getting from West Texas to the Route's starting line in Chicago, beginning with an invitation to read at the nation's longest continuously running open mic—on the Fourth of July within a national park in Arkansas. It hardly gets more American than that, and for the warm welcome we sincerely thank the hosts and audience of Wednesday Night Poetry in Hot Springs.

I took a 35mm Nikon, a souped-up MacBook, an iPhone, and a bunch of Uniballs and spiral notebooks, nothing fancier. We'd subsist on convenience-store salami and cheese when we weren't stopping to sample local roadhouse and diner fare. What a different experience it would be from the 2003 tent-camping expedition, with its array of cookpots and propane bottles, its long solo stretches, its nascent WiFi connections. In your sixties, you need more than air in your mattress.

The photographs selected for this volume are, to the greatest degree possible, contemporaneous with our 2024 journey. If an image comes from another time and trip, it'll be noted.

This is not a tourist guide, though we've written plenty of them over the years and read even more. (For our favorites, consult our handy reference guide at the back of this book.) We'd rather you think of it as a Chautauqua, in the sense that Robert Pirsig's narrator used it in *Zen and the Art of Motorcycle Maintenance.*

Muse with us about the state of the world beyond your windshield; let the road lead you into meditations on what you believe at first to be unrelated matters.

We'll often refer reverently to the Route, capitalized, as the proper personage she is: the Mother Road. But when we say "the route" generically, we mean it in the sense of the way forward, the road.

It'll be Barbara's voice you hear—the first-person "I"—through most of these paragraphs. Kay, in the passenger seat, is the sounding board, the guidebook-reader, the destination-finder, the audio-book-selector, the road-in-motion-photographer, the idea-debater. For these roles she earns her well-deserved coauthor status.

Our shared hope for the Route 66 Centennial observance is the emergence of fresh interest and pride in this national treasure. That goal seems assured already, to gauge by the plethora of websites and social media threads supplementing official resources. Further, historic preservation efforts do seem to be paying off along the Route's 2,448 miles, as the Road Ahead Partnership, the official Route 66 Centennial Commission, and state, local, and private organizations have dug in and worked diligently.

What seems less assured is a suitable civic compass for our nation as another major milestone approaches. For those who look ahead to such things, it's worth noting that the 250th birthday of the United States occurs also in 2026. Centennial celebrations for this event have also been in the works state by state, officially launching with the celebration of New Year '26 in Times Square.

As no less a thinker than author John Steinbeck pondered decades ago in *Travels with Charley: In Search of America,* how might the circuit of a country expose its shared or fractured values, for

better or for worse? We've pondered such matters as well, during our cross-country journey and numerous follow-ups.

If our responses can help reveal, can they also help heal? Turn these pages with us and join the conversation.

One regret of our Route 66 journeys in 2024 and 2025 was how many more miles of Interstate or alternate routes (see how we used that?) proved necessary due to time constraints or map miscues. It leads us to admit that it takes more than a few times to get a through-drive exactly right.

We weren't newbies to all of the Route, of course; on the contrary, there were long swaths of original pavement and Route 66 destinations familiar to us over the years. But our aim to stick perfectly to every driveable mile during three weeks of summer 2024 was thwarted more often than we'd wished. Our aim to see more must-see destinations and take more side trips was frustrated, too, by odd or unfortunate hours of arrival; and our wish to meet more of the Route's authentic residents and famed champions didn't always pan out.

To those who did accommodate our drop-in visits, phone calls, impromptu interviews, and friendly waves as we sped by, we are grateful for memories gleaned. For some it was a first acquaintance. For all, we hope it won't be the last.

Much of this content appeared first in serial form in our weekly Texas newspapers (for which we sincerely thank our longsuffering page designer Clau-

Our shared hope for the 2026 Route 66 Centennial observance is the emergence of fresh interest and pride in this national treasure.

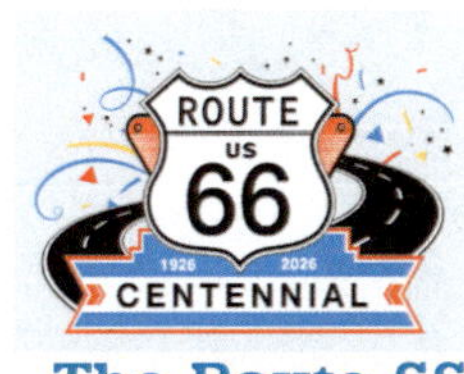

The Route 66 Centennial, 2026

The Route 66 Centennial aims to celebrate and commemorate the historic milestone of the 100th Anniversary of Route 66—and leverage it to honor the road by helping the millions who live, work, and travel along it.

In 2025, The Route 66 Road Ahead Partnership and the Route 66 Centennial Commission unveiled plans for six satellite cities to anchor the official kickoff event, which will combine a live online media event with local celebrations.

Springfield, Missouri, has been selected as the official host city for the national kickoff on April 30, 2026, at the Historic Shrine Mosque downtown and will include live entertainment, a car show, and other festivities. It will also be livestreamed globally.

The other five Satellite Cities are Joliet, Illinois; St. Louis, Missouri; Amarillo, Texas; Albuquerque, New Mexico; and Santa Monica, California.

• On April 30, 2026, "The Great Route 66 Centennial Convergence" will take place on the Santa Monica Pier.

• June 27-28, 2026: AAA Route 66 Road Fest in Tulsa, Oklahoma

• 2025: Some California towns begin celebrating early

If, like us, you're eager to learn more, visit route66centennial.org

dia Pérez) and has been adapted and expanded in this volume, in Adobe InDesign, by the authors. We hope the presentation reflects a sufficiently faithful facsimile of our road-adjacent experience that it will persuade others to get out and drive the Route for themselves. We appreciate the intelligent interventions of the Ad Hoc Writers of Lubbock, Texas, for more than a decade now.

Until you do, we heartily commend John Paget and Michael Wallis's forthcoming September 2026 remake of *Route 66: An American Odyssey* as a moving-picture alternative; either way, understand, as we do, that in any work of art the linear experience of travel is only hinted at, briefly bottled up in essence as distinctive, evocative, and ephemeral as a rare wine or precious perfume. Everyone's firsthand results along the road will differ. It *must* be driven and lived to be appreciated. Go thou and do likewise.

We welcome your feedback, and your own memories, online at www.barbarabrannon.com/blog, or at Facebook/Route66Ramble.

If you'd like to write, find us at P. O. Box 430, Spur USA 79370.

One last word of thanks, to two writers who likely do not realize how profoundly their own project informed our vision.

On a fortuitous evening in the Black Hills during Western Writers of America 2023 we listened, rapt, to Texan karla k morton and her fellow-traveler, Alan Birkelbach, as they described their travels and travails during a year-long circuit of America's national parks. Yes, *all* of them. Theirs was not a through-trip for the faint of heart, but it was perfectly suited to a pair of poets. We honor and emulate their passion for adventure and their understanding of what makes a place worth visiting: to tell *its* story as much as to tell yours.

Barbara Brannon
Spur, Texas • January 2026

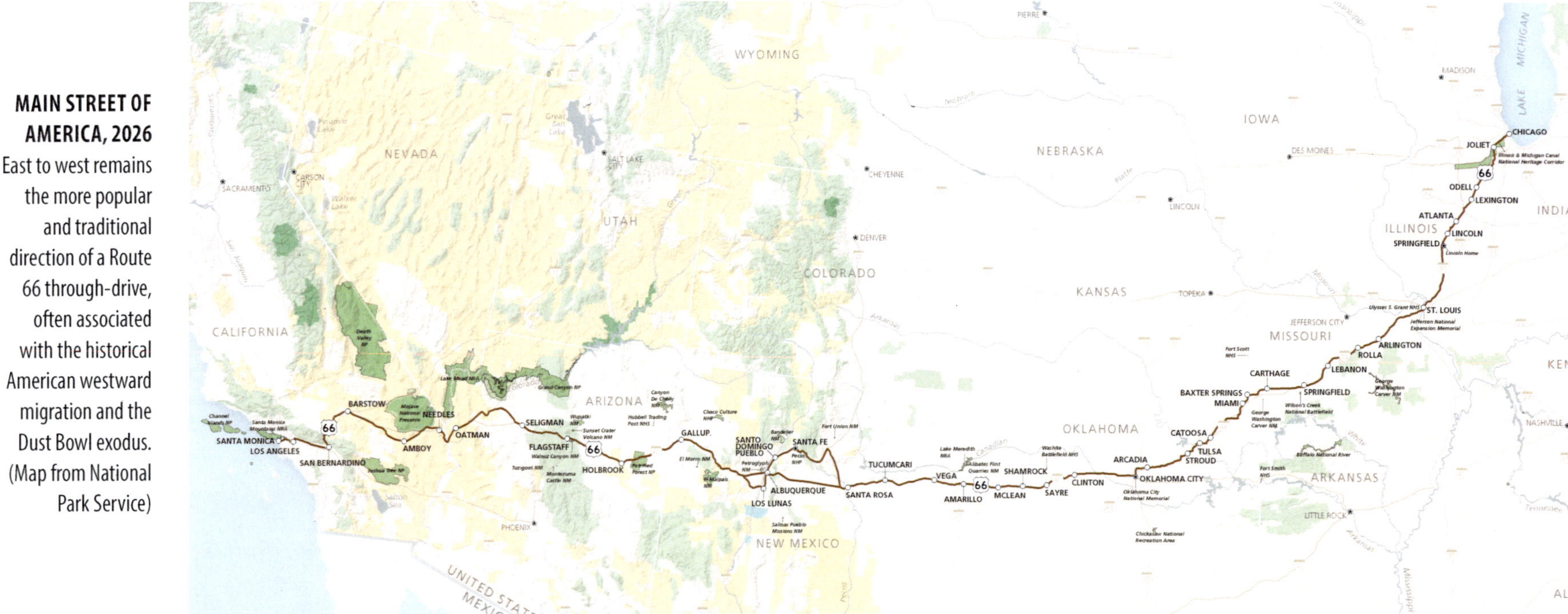

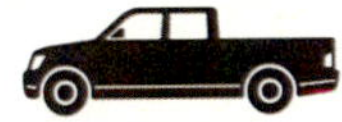

Burgaw to Barstow, 2003

Our first experience of Route 66 has been more than two decades ago now.

Back then we lived in Wilmington, North Carolina, where, just outside the gates of the university where I taught there was an inconspicuous but curious mileage sign at the outset of westbound I-40.

"Barstow, Calif. 2,554." (It was there in 2003 when this photo was taken; it was stolen; it was replaced and stolen again—and finally, replaced and made more permanent.)

Locals would wonder what the California end looked like. They'd sometimes comment on the odd feeling of connectedness it gives them when they drive past it. They'd get to thinking about anecdotes from the highway's history, or recount what it was like to travel to the the coast here before the Interstate. They'd talk about how the road has brought change, and lots of newcomers, to their small town.

So that June I set out solo—on the anniversary date of the completion of I-40 to its Wilmington terminus—to check it all out for myself.

I pitched the idea of a serial travelogue to our newspaper, the *Wilmington Star-News,* and back in the era of limited Internet the editors helped me work out a system for filing a story and photos at the end of each day's travel, wherever I might camp for the night. They included a map of my progress and listed an AOL address where readers could send me their own suggestions and stories along the way.

The paper billed it "Burgaw to Barstow: One Woman. One Road. And It All Began With a Single Sign."

Starting at Oklahoma City the magnet of Route 66 pavement drew me, often, from the high-speed divided highway onto the old road it had displaced. I heard the stories of ghost towns, shuttered cafes, abandoned gas stations. "They done killed the Mother Road," one shopkeeper said, recalling the year her parents were forced to shut down their motor court in Shamrock, Texas.

Kay flew out to join me at a few points. We saw the Texas outdoor musical and the Cadillac Ranch, legends we'd later claim as part of home.

Across most of the West landmarks of the "Get Your Kicks" era lay fallow and sad, decrepit, abandoned. The vestiges of old 66 had to be diligently searched out.

It wasn't long afterwards that salvation arrived like a bolt of lightning—Lightning McQueen of the 2006 *Cars* animated film, that is. The movie brought the Mother Road back to life, largely thanks to the participation of Route champion Michael Wallis, who ensured authenticity at every turn, and Pixar's John Lasseter, whose imagination brought joy at every turn. Suddenly, Route 66 was cool again.

By the time we'd relocated to Texas, a movement was taking root to document and preserve stretches of original pavement, and contributing structures. A National Parks study in 1990 and a federal Route 66 Corridor Preservation Program in 2000 invited community input throughout all eight Route 66 states. Brown signage and pavement stencils appeared, little by little. The Road was on its way to a full-blown centennial celebration for 2026. It only remains to see a Route 66 National Historic Trail Designation Act signed into law at last—still not a done deal at the time of this writing.

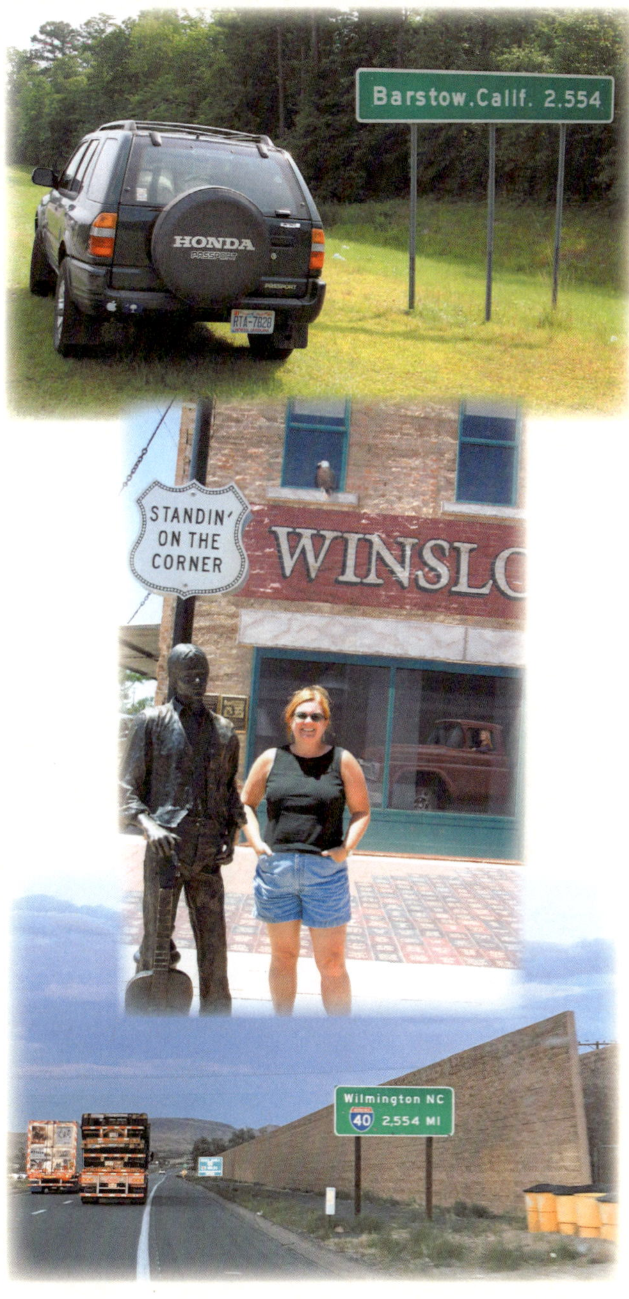

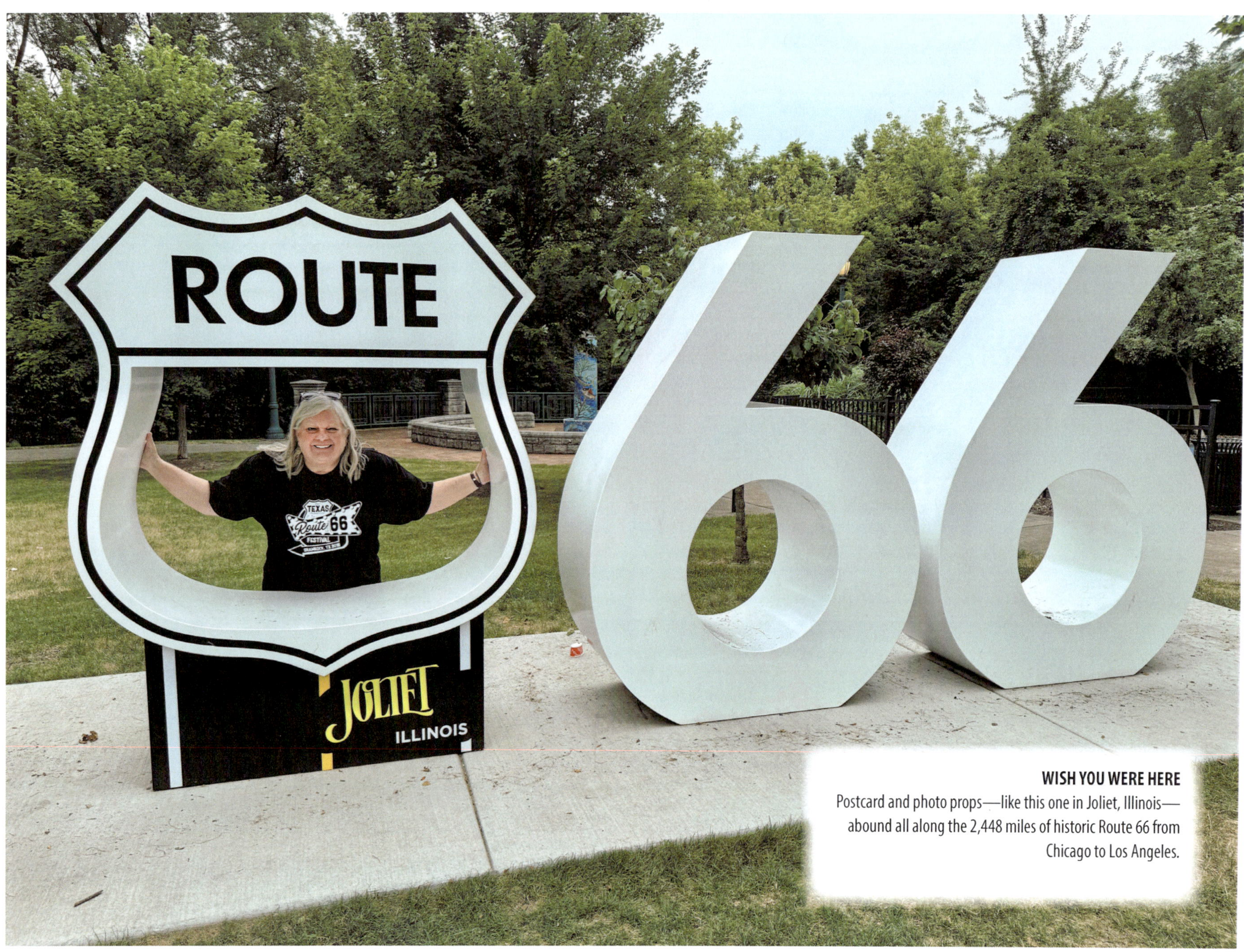

WISH YOU WERE HERE
Postcard and photo props—like this one in Joliet, Illinois—abound all along the 2,448 miles of historic Route 66 from Chicago to Los Angeles.

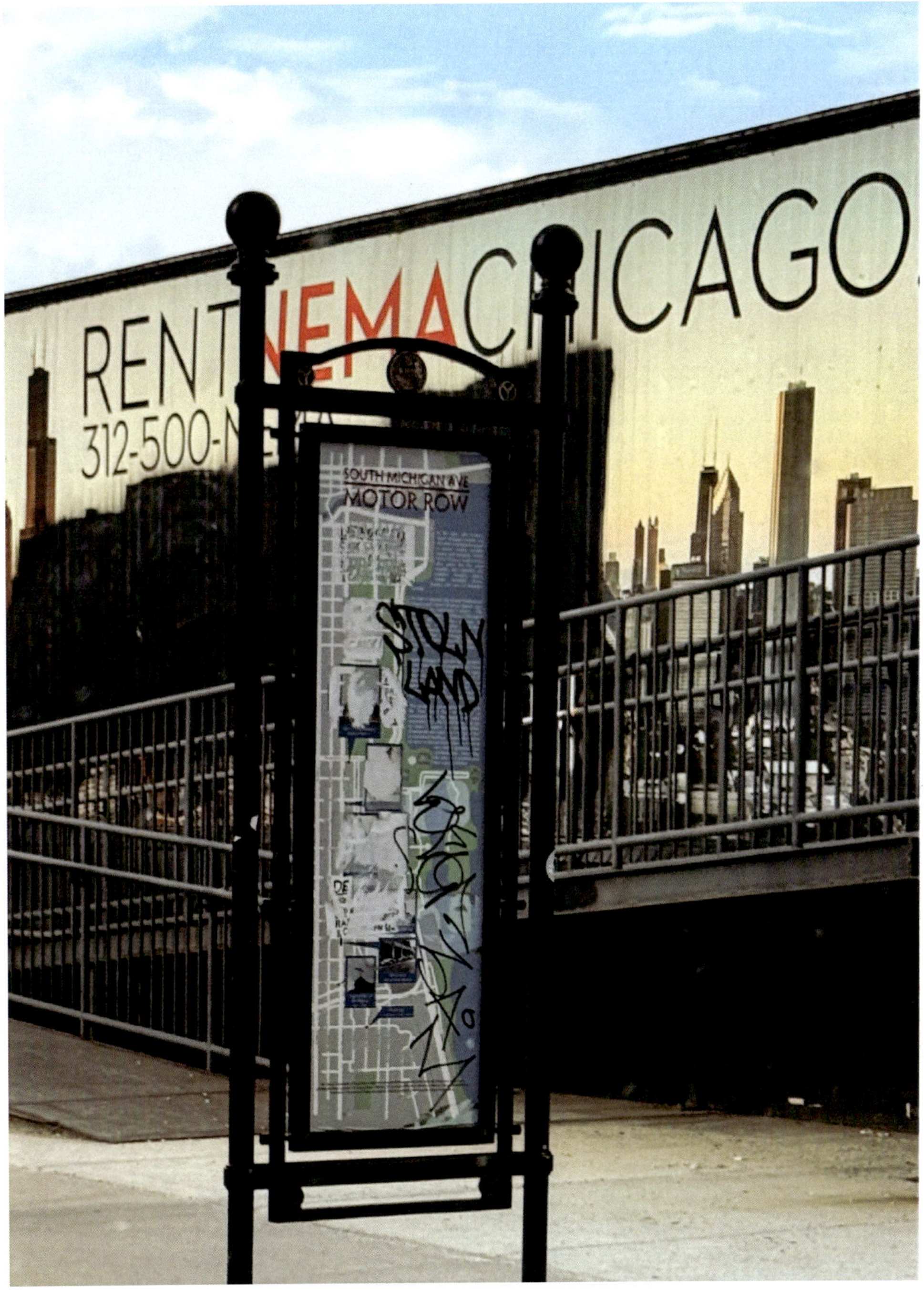

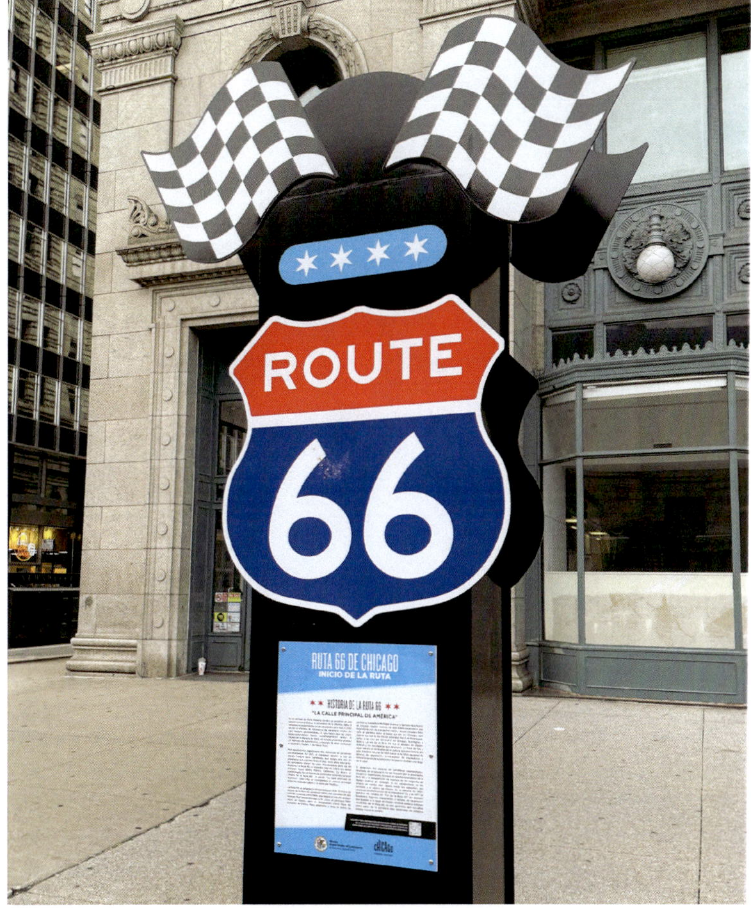

SIGN, SIGN This colorful new sign above helps Route 66 travelers mark their starting line along busy Michigan Avenue across the street from the Art Institute of Chicago. A year later, as we saw on social media, the signage had, regrettably been plastered over by hundreds of visitors' stickers.

STOLN CHICAGOLAND Any human-made sign, it seems, is a mark of one people's colonization: if numbered shields help drivers safely navigate terrain that a society has claimed for its own and civilized, what's to prevent earlier inhabitants from using others' wayfinding aids as reminders? From the outset of our journey this graffiti made us mindful that our track overlaid those of countless others.

In search of the Mother Road

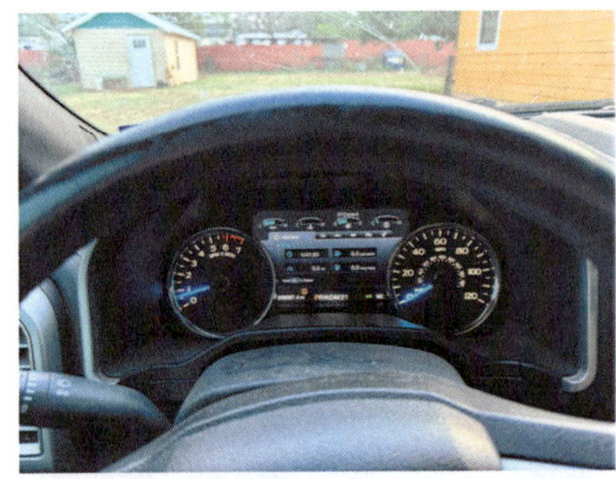

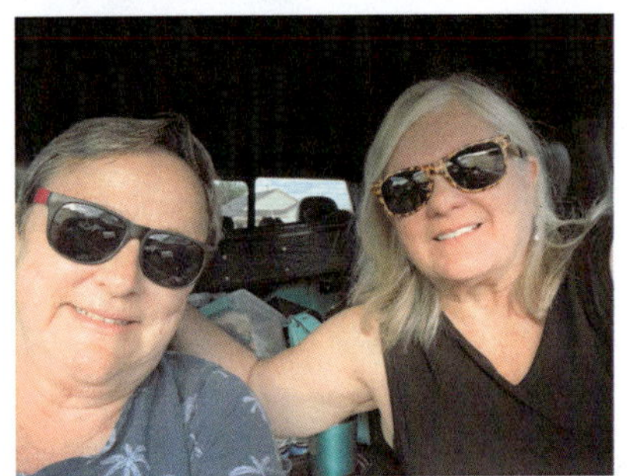

SPURRED ON A JOURNEY Driving our redoubtable Black Beauty Ford F150, we first made our way from home in Spur, Texas, to Chicago, Illinois.

It's rare that local newspaper editors—especially ones like us, who have an active stake in hometown publications that go to press once a week year round—get to take an extended vacation. No Caribbean cruises or gala getaways for us.

Yet our comparative freedom to report from the road does provide some unique opportunities for perspective, whenever we can sync travel with deadlines.

Given the fractious state of our national consciousness these days, along with simple curiosity as a couple of important American anniversaries approached in 2026, at the height of summer two writers itched to get out and see a few things for ourselves.

Kay and I saw an opening in the calendar with sufficient time and resources to drive across the country's heartland. Though we'd been based in West Texas for nearly two decades (and one half of our team was born and raised here), there was still a whole lot more of our country to see to the left of us.

Starting out on the eve of America's birthday, we got ourselves in due time from Texas to Chicago, our Mile Zero. We'd kicked off our trip in a national park in Arkansas on the eve of July 4, at a writers' gathering. Organizers made it a safe space for people of all cultures, all persuasions, and all nationalities. Two visitors were collecting signatures to get a reproductive freedom initiative on the ballot. Readers of all skin colors had signed up. The host opened with a recitation, raising her hand in a pose we all recognized, of "The New Colossus" by Emma Lazarus. Now *this* was how to start a vacation!

A few days later we reached the starting gate on Chicago's Michigan Avenue. We had a ways to go: some 2,448 miles at minimum.

If you've ever listened to the famous song, any version from that first Nat King Cole rendition to the Texas take by Ray Benson and Asleep at the Wheel, you already know where I'm going with this.

If you e-ver plan to mo-tor west . . . Get your kicks—on Route Sixty-Six.

Visions of tailfin convertibles, neon signs, sleeping in an ersatz teepee might spring to mind. We'd do our best to find those. Streams and rivers spanned by two-lane arched

> *Visions of tailfin convertibles, neon signs, sleeping in a teepee might spring to mind …we also wanted to get a handle on what makes our nation tick, or not.*

bridges, old-style milk shakes, mom-and-pop motor courts, giant roadside statues. Tales told by old-timers. And that legendary highway shield with its magical double digits.

But like John Steinbeck in his 1962 opus *Travels with Charley: In Search of America,* we also wanted to get a handle on what makes our nation tick, or not. Steinbeck, who had himself provided Route 66's most famous nickname, "The Mother Road," in his 1939 Pulitzer Prize–winning *The Grapes of Wrath,* set out to learn what people in all corners of the country felt and thought in the midst of a global nuclear stalemate, a race to space, and a time-bomb of racial tension. He took a poodle for company.

Not considering cats companionable for travel, Kay and I left ours home at the newspaper office and took each other.

We reset the trip meter upon finding the Begin Historic Route 66 marker at Michigan and Adams, as so many travelers before us have done. Our Rocinante would be a 2015 half-ton Ford pickup nicknamed Black Beauty. She'd seen us through any number of adventures already. She was outfitted, like Steinbeck's rig, with a high-capacity fuel tank, tools we hoped not to need, and too many books.

It was a beautiful evening on the Lake Michigan shore, with summer revelers taking in a music festival in Grant Park, riding the Navy Pier Ferris wheel, enjoying a hot dog, or simply cruising the Route. Navigating the mighty multi-lane traffic, we struggled to follow the trail of brown signs.

Today, much of the 1926 (and later) blacktop of Route 66 has long since been paved over, moved, or obliterated altogether. The legendary highway that once funneled freight traffic and fun-seekers westward, or delivered desperate families from the Dust Bowl to a more hopeful home in California, was subsumed bit by bit by wider and straighter throughways. Its original alignments through the hearts of small downtowns lined by brick storefronts, cafés, and newfangled service stations gave way to bypasses and eventually to the inexorable juggernaut of the Interstates. In 1985 the route made famous in song and story was decommissioned altogether.

"Excessive truck use during World War II and the comeback of the automobile industry immediately following the war brought great pressure to bear

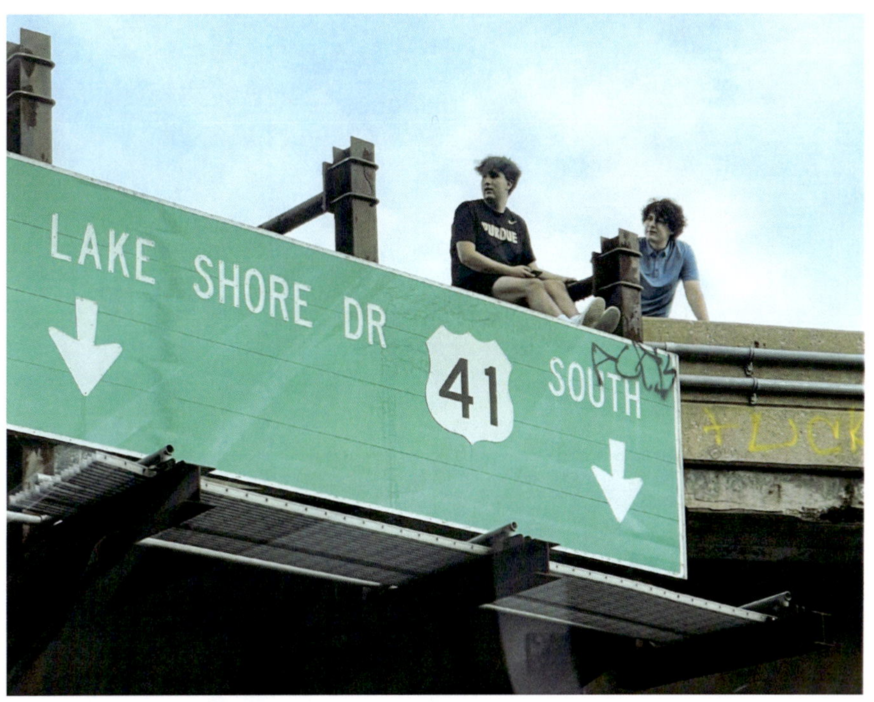

GETTING TO THE ROUTE there's no telling what sights you'll see—or from which viewpoints.

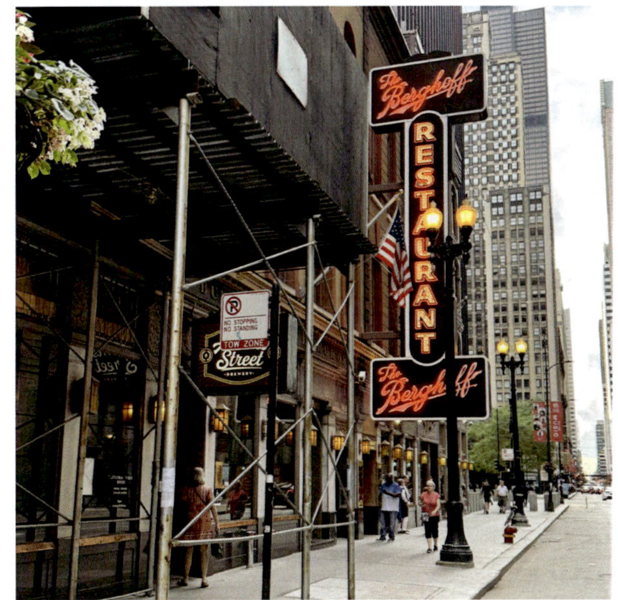

BERGHOFF'S RESTAURANT on the Chicago Loop—only steps from the starting point of Route 66—has been family-operated for more than 125 years.

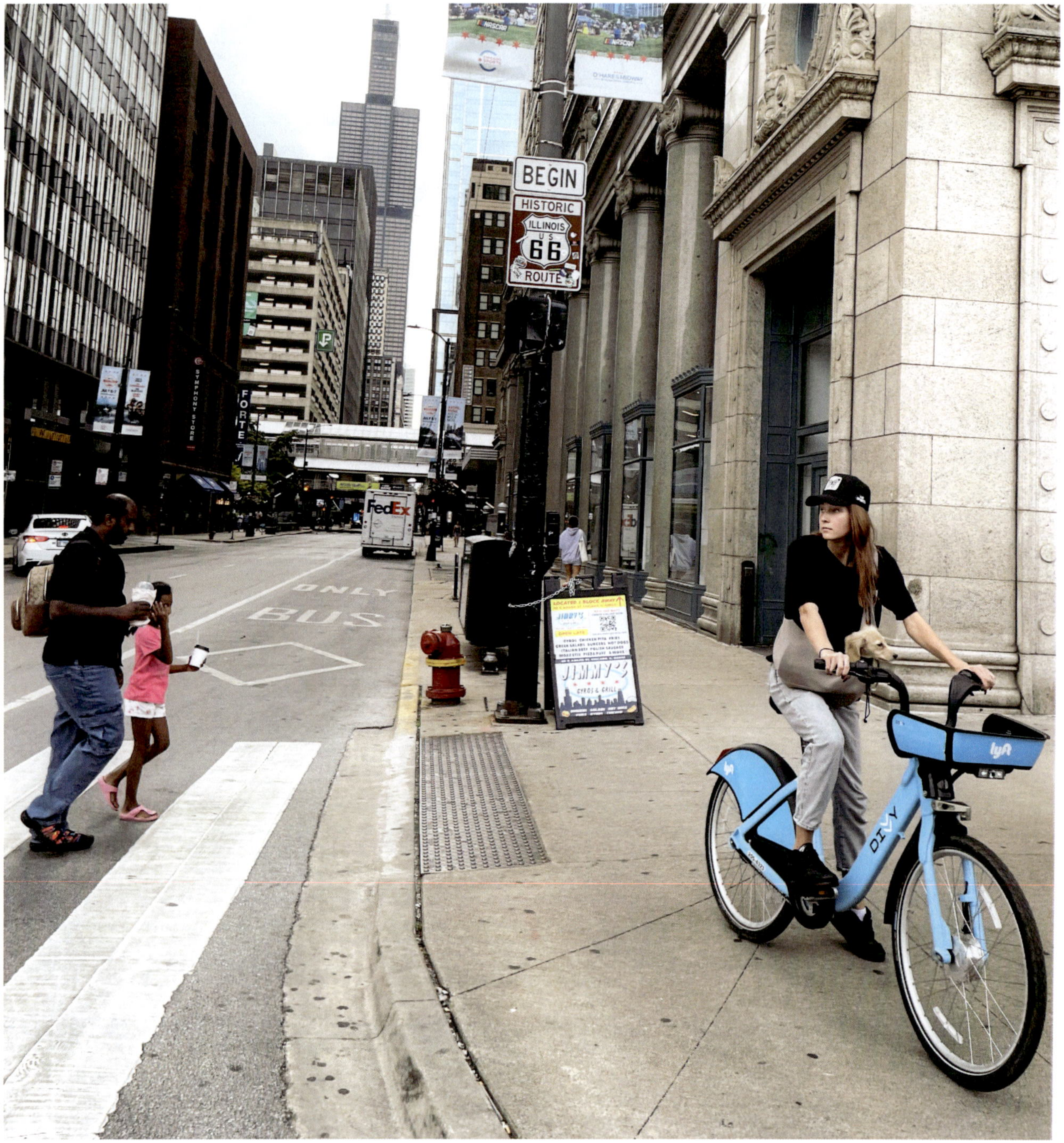

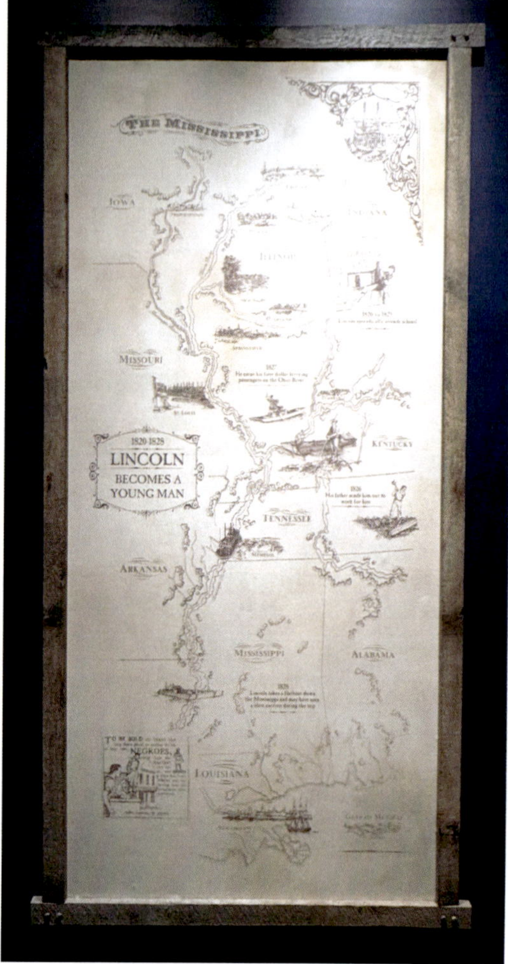

EVERYWHERE A SIGN Following the 2,448 miles (give or take a few, depending on which routing you take), brown-and-white official signs mark different alignments of Route 66 over different periods of the road's history. Sometimes stretches of original, or at least older, pavement exist; in other places, original road was torn up, blocked off, or overpaved by other highways. A map is a must; one of the best is Jerry McClanahan's *Route 66 EZ 66 Guide for Travelers*, now in its 5th edition (visit www.national66.org).

on America's highways," reads a page on the U.S. National Park Service's informational website ("Demise and Resurgence of Interest in Route 66"). "Automobile production jumped from just over 65,000 cars in 1945 to 3.9 million in 1948. Meanwhile, the deterioration of the national highway system was appalling. Virtually all roads, including Route 66, were functionally obsolete because of narrow pavements and antiquated structural features that reduced carrying capacity."

But by the century's last decade the Route 66 Study Act of 1990, recognizing that the Mother Road had "become a symbol of the American people's heritage of travel and their legacy of seeking a better life," paved the way for restoration of some segments. A resurgence of interest by preservation and heritage tourism groups (such as the one by which I was employed soon afterward) led to historical waymarking, interpretation, and economic development incentives.

Those efforts, boosted by the Disney/Pixar *Cars* animated film phenomenon in 2006, got the traffic flowing again. Today, an estimated 85 percent of the old route is driveable in some form. It's hard to even get a grasp on the numbers of leisure travelers from around the U.S. and the world who choose Route 66 as a "destination." The economic benefit to local businesses is staggering.

Yet does the linear bubble of Route 66 accurately reflect the temper of the country in tempestuous times? We weren't sure.

On the day we departed Chicago, the *Sun-Times* newspaper reported twenty-one people killed and at least 84 others wounded by gunfire in the city during the extended Fourth of July weekend. By the time we'd reached Tucumcari, New Mexico, at the end of the week, the nation was rocked by news of an assassination attempt on a once and future president. Animosities personal and political continued to threaten our nation, it was regrettably clear.

Fiery words, firearms, and firebrands. Are the divisions they signal greater, or lesser, than in the roiled-up nation President Abraham Lincoln faced when elected to its highest office in November 1860? Only six weeks afterward, Southern states began seceding from the Union. To understand the temper of America in those dark days, we'd be spending some time among the exhibits at the Lincoln Presidential Library and Museum in the Illinois capital of Springfield.

Our mission became to take our readers there, and to every state along the way west to the Pacific. We determined we would try to put our fingers on the pulse, take the temperature, figure out what makes Route 66 tick…what makes America tick.

Whatever metaphor you prefer, the Mother Road continues to roll out the panorama of American experience in a fashion unlike any other. She guides us to witness and appreciate the westering urge of those who have gone before; to explore the changing terrain and evolving mindsets of those who inhabit it; to delve deep into our collective impulses to conquer and claim.

The perspective is illuminating. ☞

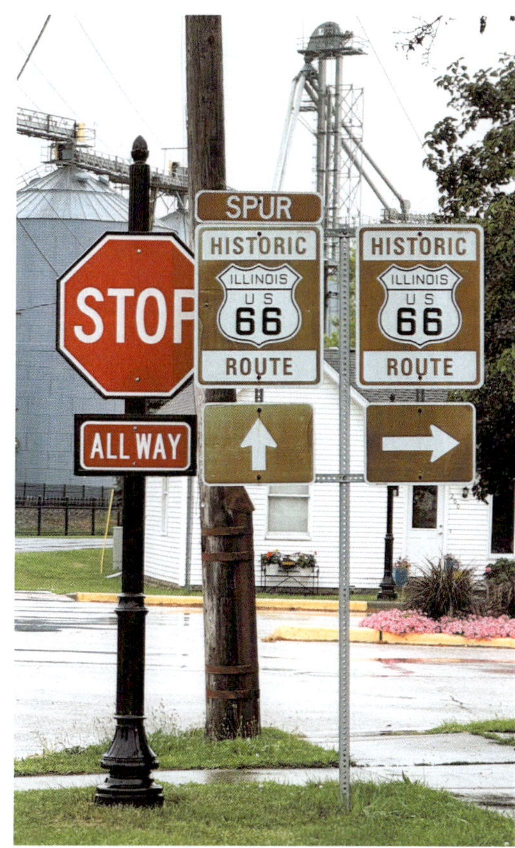

IN ILLINOIS most Route 66 signs point north and south. The Abraham Lincoln Presidential Museum and Library — also a great place for writing while enjoying a bite of lunch in the cafe — are located in Springfield, the state's capital. Lincoln's spirit lighted our way and set a tone for thinking about our nation.

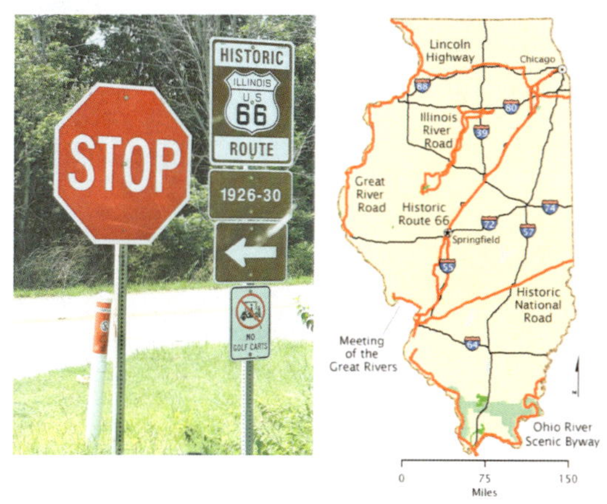

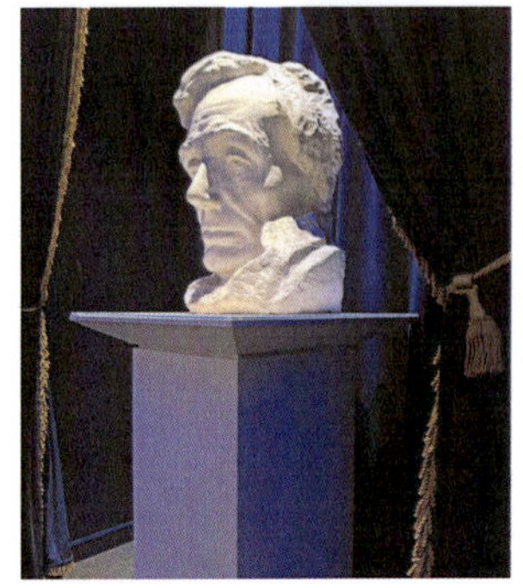
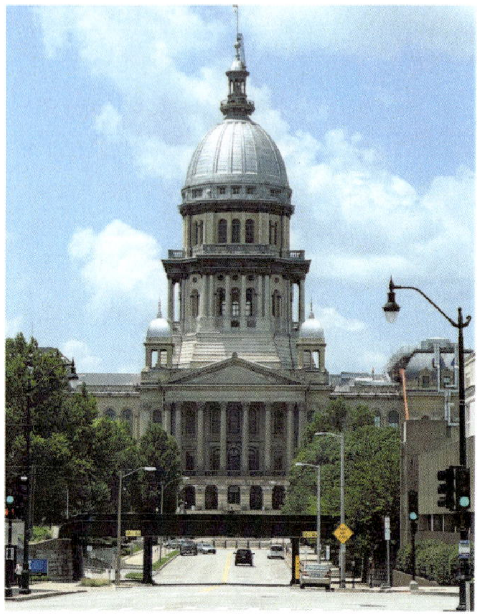

CHAPTER ONE
Route 66 in the Land of Lincoln

"THE ROAD AHEAD" IS THE TITLE of the preservation partnership that has worked since 2018 to designate Route 66 a National Historic Trail, under the leadership of Bill Thomas of Atlanta, Illinois. After a quick reconnection with him at the town's newly opened American Giants Museum, we pulled out in a pouring rainstorm, continuing toward California in the only state where the westward-inclined Mother Road runs north-south.

"I'm confident Rt. 66 will become our country's newest National Historic Trail soon, and look forward to continuing to work to achieve that goal," Thomas wrote in the organization's quarterly report posted shortly before our meeting. Representatives in the eight Route 66 states had signed onto a House bill to that effect, reintroduced in June 2023. But while Congress has taken important steps, the measure is hardly moving at Lightning McQueen speed—and has yet to cross the finish line.

In 2022, U.S. senators Ted Cruz of Texas and others introduced a companion Senate bill. As of this writing it's still sitting in committee, with the 2026 anniversary of the Mother Road fast approaching.

> *"Route 66 has fueled America's imagination, popular culture, and passion for the open road for nearly a century. It deserves a place not just in our rearview mirror, but on our roadmap of unique travel experiences for generations to come."*
> *— Stephanie Meeks, former president and CEO of the National Trust for Historic Preservation*

As our tires touch as much of the original road ("alignment," in highway terms) as still exists, we can readily appreciate the enormous economic benefit that communities of all sizes realize from the throngs who drive some portion of it annually. More than a dozen years ago the pioneering Rutgers study conservatively estimated the total U.S. impact at $132 million annually.

But divisiveness and stalemates are nothing new in our federal government, as current events show, and as we appreciated even more profoundly during our visit to one Route 66 site in particular: the Abraham Lincoln Presidential Museum and Library in Springfield, capital of Illinois.

The conundrums our nation's 16th president faced over states' rights versus federal authority during his first election campaign are clarified through documents (approximately 12 million of them, dating as far back as the 18th century, with a small selection of facsimiles on display in the library's entry lobby) and interpretive exhibits (enough to easily fill half a day's sojourn in the museum).

The story of Lincoln's rise from an "undistinguished" family and humble

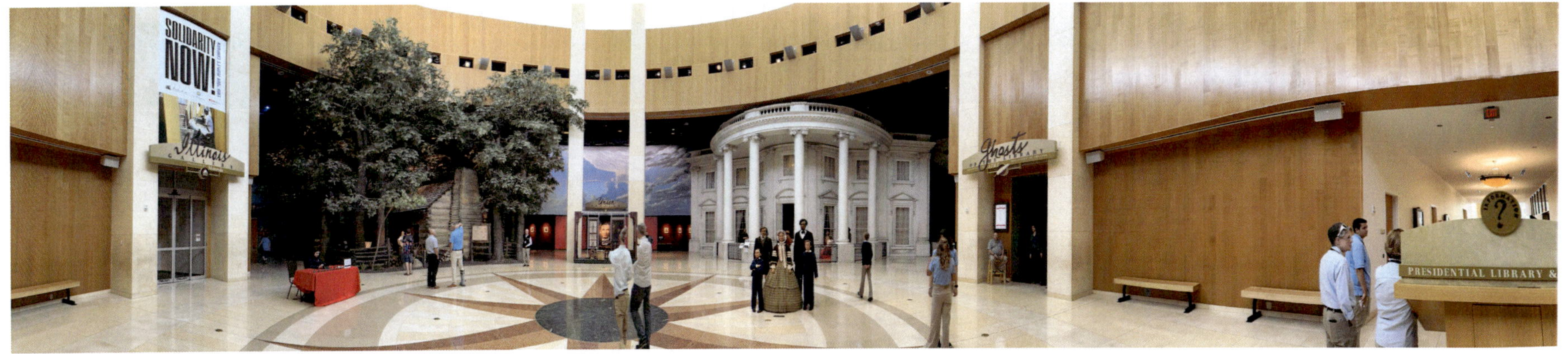

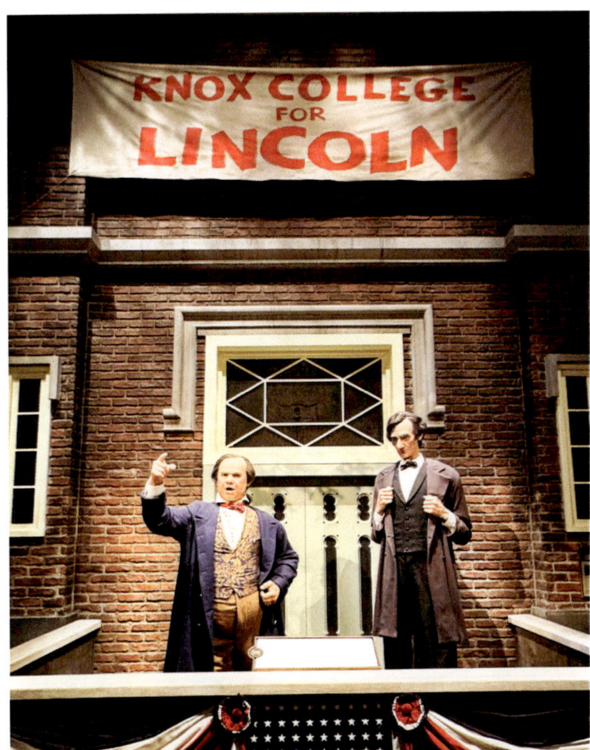

KNOX COLLEGE
FOR
LINCOLN

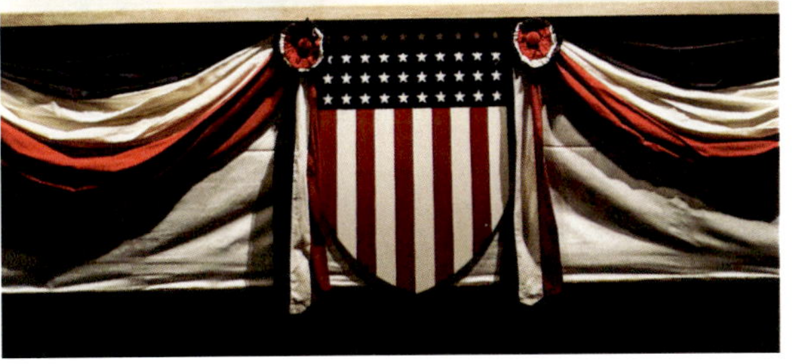

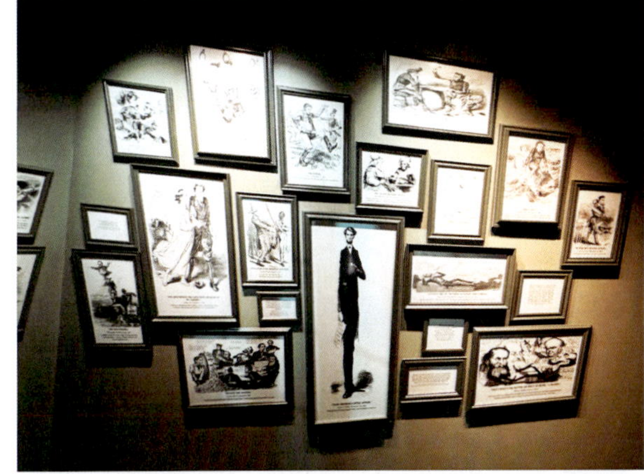

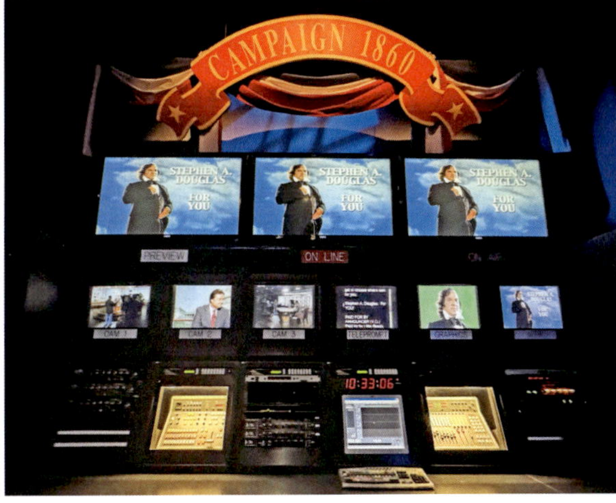

CAMPAIGN 1860
STEPHEN A. DOUGLAS
FOR YOU
PREVIEW
ON LINE
ON AIR

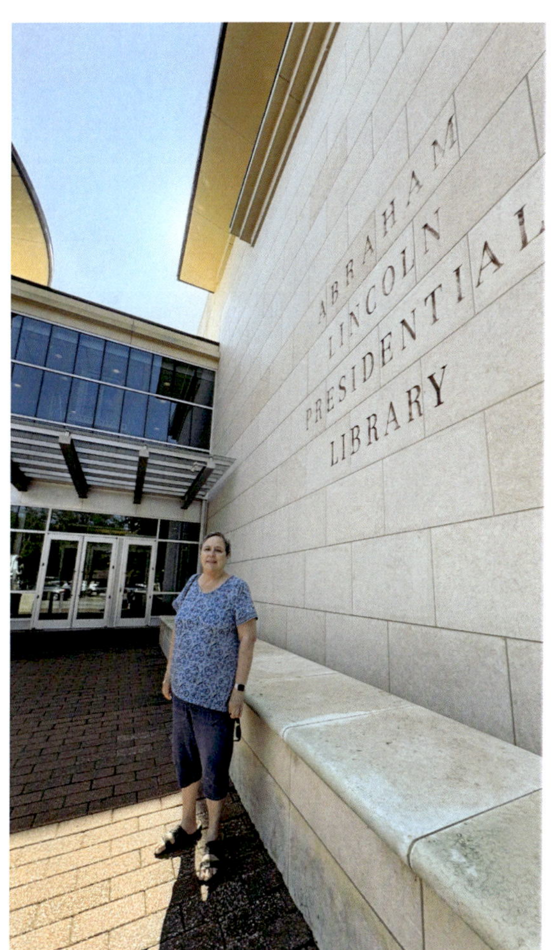

ABRAHAM
LINCOLN
PRESIDENTIAL
LIBRARY

roots to a skilled militiaman, self-educated lawyer, and devoted family man—and ultimately to the White House—is presented in a variety of clever exhibits.

The interpretation of Lincoln's family life, his political career, the U.S. amid civil war, and his assassination and aftermath all richly augmented our learning. From lifelike dioramas to reproductions of images and letters, to a Holovision theater experience, to a walk-through reproduction of the White House of the 1860s, each aspect of Lincoln's life and career is brought into context.

Forensics students looking to understand the premise of a current-day Lincoln-Douglas Debate, researchers grappling to understand the evolving front—and rising casualties—of the War Between the States, or cultural historians interested in the fashions of the day might all find fresh insights.

But most telling, to me, were the reproductions of political screeds and cartoons of Lincoln's time. Scores of these are skewed in off-kilter frames, hung in exhibit spaces of wildly distorted walls and doors, to echo the cant of critics' biting words and images.

By comparison, today's news media might come off as polite as greeting cards. More akin to the 19th-century voices depicted here is the 21st-century's social media space, or its often obscene flags and bumper stickers—a healthy dose of which we noted along the road in every state. I mused on these matters as I wondered whether history is, as claimed, doomed to repeat itself.

But the Lincoln museum has a lot to teach with regard to hope for a strong American union. Once re-fused during an arduous Reconstruction, as the exhibits also cover, the states proved resilient and, at intervals, forward-thinking. A temporary exhibition highlighted more recent struggles for civil rights—reminding us pointedly that the work is far from over.

Inspired by words and acts of greatness, I composed most of this chapter within that powerfully evocative space. Like the home and the tomb we had visited the evening prior, it is a place both uplifting and humbling, joyful and sobering.

As we hit the road again that afternoon, I was ready to appreciate, afresh, a pavement that once knit together a growing number of states, some acquired by arm-twisting deals, some as new as Oklahoma and Arizona (which didn't become a part of the Union until 1907 and 1912 respectively), one (Texas) that had even been a sovereign nation.

Historic preservation, economic benefit, and open-road vacations are all great reasons to appreciate the treasure that is Route 66. But so are the lessons the Route can teach us about what it means to be American. 🖘

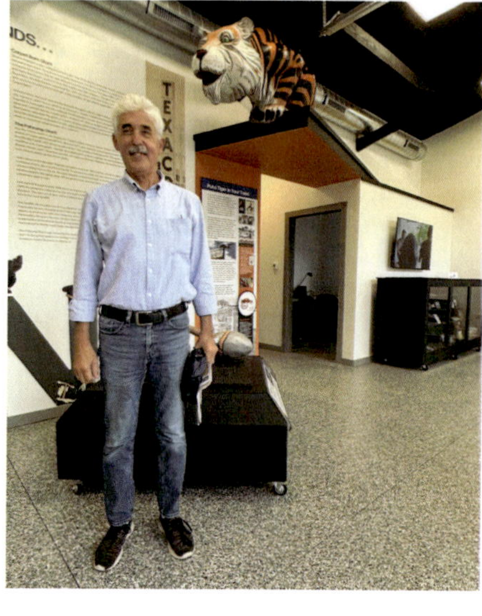

ROUTE WARRIOR AMONG GIANTS
Route champion and former schoolteacher Bill Thomas of Atlanta, Illinois, chair of the Route 66 Road Ahead Partnership, was named in 2022 to the national Route 66 Centennial Commission. The group has been coordinating ways to observe, promote, and benefit from 100 years of the Route in 2026.

IN ATLANTA, ILLINOIS (one of 19 Atlantas in the U.S., and which just happens to be named for Barbara's Georgia hometown), the newly opened American Giants museum tells the story of roadside advertising figures from Muffler Men to Paul Bunyan, to Big Boy and the Esso Tiger. Photo ops abound; and in the two years since our trip there, many more fiberglass giants have congregated at the site.

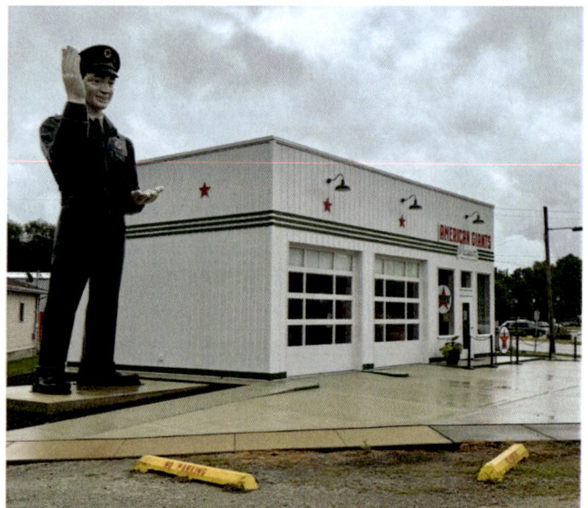

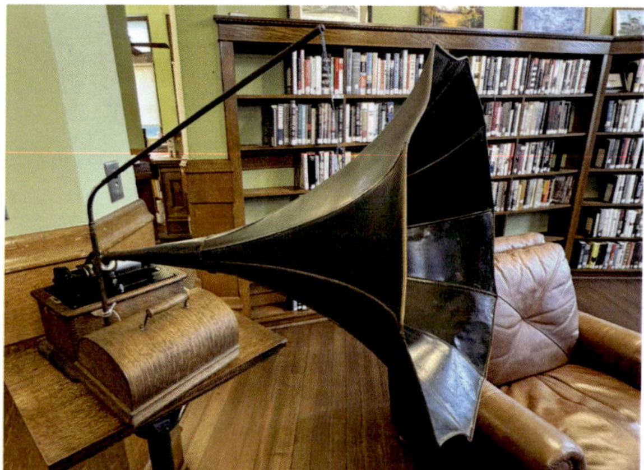

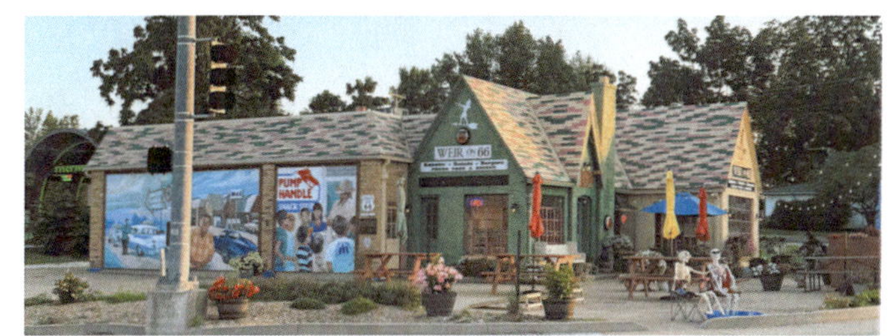

WEIR OPEN In 1932, Paul T. Carr built the old Phillips 66 station in Cuba, Missouri, which also served as a site for used car sales; later it housed the Wallis Oil Company, in the 20th century it was restored as a café.

Show Me 'Mo' of Missouri

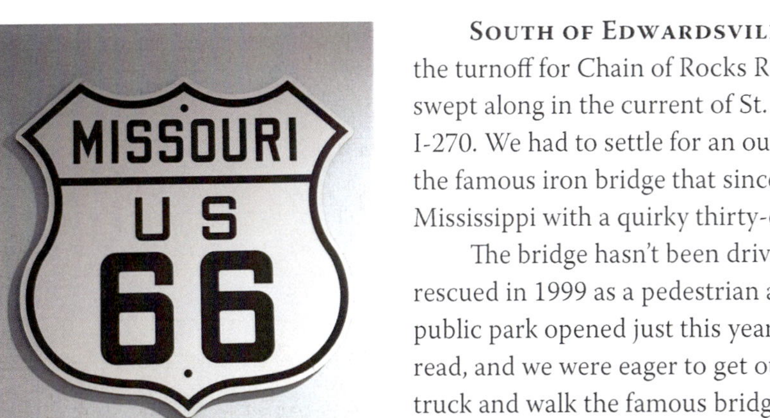

YOU GO THROUGH SAINT LOOEY and Joplin, Missouri—according to "Route 66" songwriter Bobby Troup—following this famous shield.

SOUTH OF EDWARDSVILLE, ILLINOIS, in search of the turnoff for Chain of Rocks Road, we wound up instead swept along in the current of St. Louis–bound trucks on I-270. We had to settle for an out-the-window view of the famous iron bridge that since 1927 has spanned the Mississippi with a quirky thirty-degree bend in the middle.

The bridge hasn't been drivable since 1968, but it was rescued in 1999 as a pedestrian and bicycle route. A new public park opened just this year on the St. Louis side, we'd read, and we were eager to get out of the truck and walk the famous bridge for the views and the exercise.

Alas, as was to prove the case often in the days to come, the contradictions of paper map, digital map and road signs foiled our best attempts to stick to existing old-route pavement. If I had taken good advice weeks ago and mail-ordered the set of eight acclaimed Ross/McClanahan "Here It Is!" maps, we'd have saved some grief in wayfinding. Jerry McClanahan's spiral-bound *EZ 66 Guide for Travelers* (which we acquired from a bookstore later on our journey) is a good compromise, but it's so chock-full of detail that a capable and patient navigator in the copilot's

seat is a must. By this I mean one who isn't prone to dozing on boring stretches.

The digital maps we've come to rely on daily in the iPhone age aren't up to the task of locating Old Route 66, and in my recent experience, the plethora of other mobile apps aren't, either. For those who are inclined to rely on turn-by-turn guidance (this subset does *not* include me), there's an *EZ Guide* version (the "Yellow App") for that, but we hadn't road-tested it before departure.

> *A capable and patient navigator in the copilot's seat is a must. By this I mean one who isn't prone to dozing on boring stretches.*

Having also been foiled on the Missouri side of the big river by construction closure of the cloverleaf leading to the new Chain of Rocks Park, we prepared to embrace everything else the Show Me State had to offer.

Neither Kay nor I were familiar with Missouri. I barely recalled my cross-country traverse by bus in the centennial year of 1976 when the Gateway Arch flickered by as if in a home-movie reel. Now I wanted to see this door to the West up close and to appreciate how modernist architect Eero Saarinen's design became as much an icon of St. Louis as the Space Needle, the Statue of Liberty or the Eiffel Tower have become for their cities.

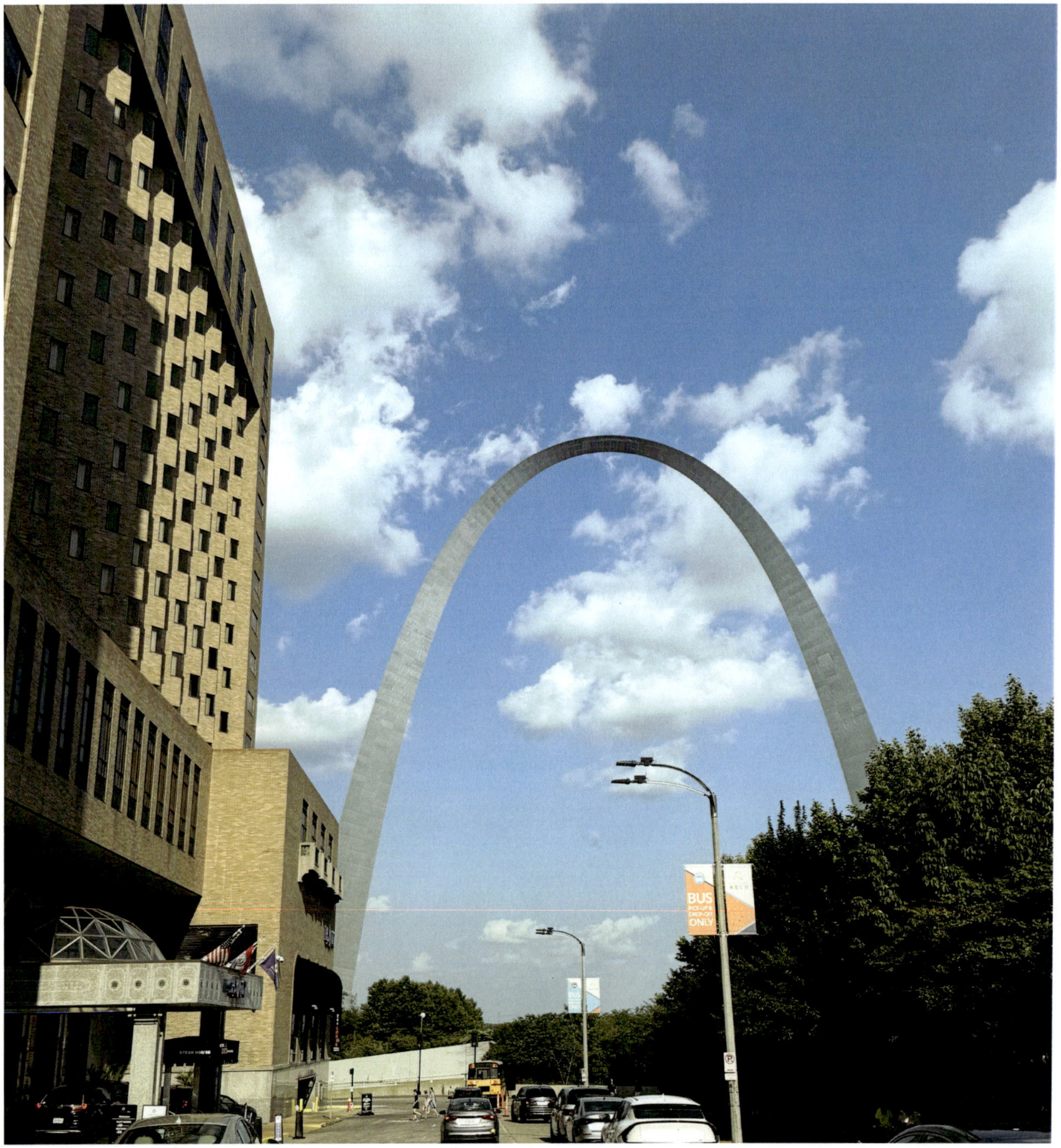

RISING 630 FEET over the St. Louis skyline and overlooking the Mississippi River a few miles south of its confluence with the Missouri, the Gateway Arch serves as symbol of the city—and exploration of the American West.

CARDINAL NUMBERS flocked to Busch Stadium for a Wednesday night baseball game (the hometown Cards, however, lost to the Kansas City Royals, 6–4).

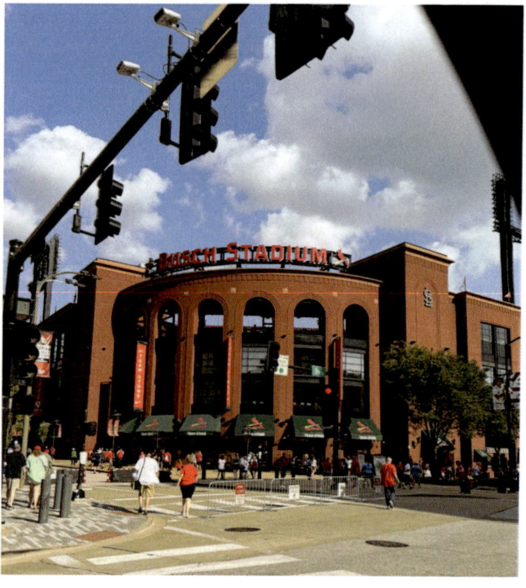

The site's National Park Service website provides useful background for the 1965 icon. "Neither an obelisk nor a rectangular box nor a dome seemed right on this site or for this purpose," Saarinen wrote. "But here, at the edge of the Mississippi River, a great arch did seem right."

And it does.

Gleaming in the vesper sunlight as we approach it from the bluffs of Riverview Drive and the bricked vista of Florissant Avenue, the Arch seems to beckon those on the opposite bank to join us in this grand adventure. I recall the previous summer tracking Lewis and Clark's Corps of Discovery, far up on the mighty Missouri. I'd begun to wrap my head around the vastness of this continent when it was wilderness. Some say untamed; I say un*claimed,* except by tribes who needed no metes and bounds, no Google Maps to define their territories, and have had to exercise determination to retain or reclaim them.

I take a deep breath as we pause in one traffic-less moment in the lee of the shining Arch. Full of that promise of the West, we're ready to light out for California.

Between us and Joplin, clear on the other side of the state, there are a lot of Missouri hills and woods. Wikipedia tells us that the etymological origin of "Ozarks" might be the French *aux arcs*—"land of the arches"—recalling natural rock bridges formed by erosion and collapsed caves in the region. We'll go with that, as the green land rolls like a magic carpet beneath our Rocinante.

Among the region's destination "show caves," Meramec Caverns beckons like a carnival barker from manifold billboards and barn signs. Part of its Route 66 lore is that the flashy Lester Benton Dill, who opened it as a tourist attraction back in the 1930s, began gluing promotional cards to car bumpers (also a recent development) while visitors were inside exploring his caves. A decade or so later, when adhesive plastic was invented, the bumper sticker, well, stuck.

If the bumper sticker and the billboard became the magnets to draw in visitors' dollars along tourist routes, these days what keeps them staying longer and spending more is the building mural.

Whether an early-era advertising message colorfully painted on crumbling brick (and often remaining dimly visible a century later as a "ghost" sign) or a newly crafted artwork embodying local symbolism, the mural has

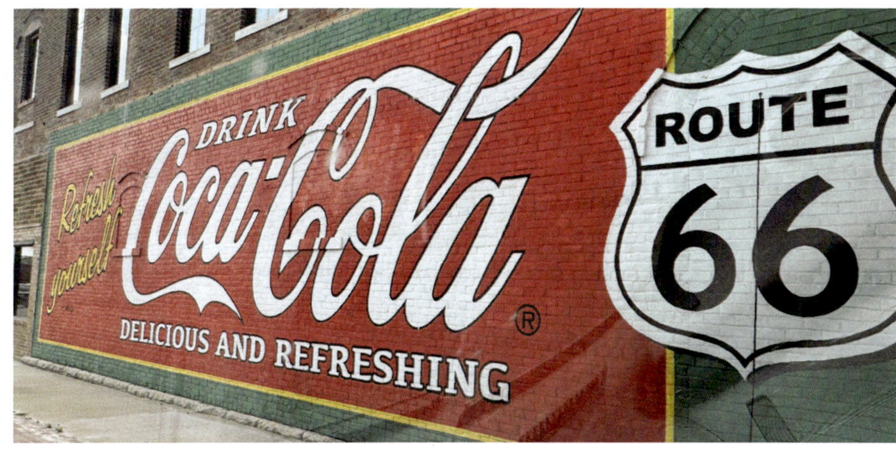

COCA-COLA wasn't as prevalent in the midwestern part of the U.S., where we found that often Pepsi products dominated in restaurants and soda fountains—at least in 2024.

emerged as a proven mechanism for town pride and traveler engagement. Not to mention the much-needed income commissions provide to hungry artists.

If the Mother Road had a birthplace as well as a starting point, it's Springfield, Missouri, by virtue of hosting the highway association meeting at which it was granted its memorable number, thanks to highway advocates Cyrus Avery and John T. Woodruff. The auspicious event occurred on April 30, 1926. (A hundred years to the day, America's Route 66 Centennial Celebration would kick off there, we'd later learn.)

Full of that promise of the West, we're ready to light out for California.

Joplin, tucked into the southwest corner of Missouri (and the largest city in the Four State Area of Oklahoma, Arkansas, Missouri, and Kansas), was a mining boomtown in the 19th century. A bustling downtown center and fine neighborhoods blossomed by the 1920s, but that didn't erase something of a wild-and-woolly reputation.

"In 1933 during the Great Depression," saith our handy digital source, Wikipedia, "the notorious criminals Bonnie and Clyde spent some weeks in Joplin, where they robbed several area businesses. Tipped off by a neighbor, the Joplin Police Department attempted to apprehend the pair. Bonnie and Clyde escaped after killing Newton County Constable John Wesley Harryman and Joplin Police Detective Harry McGinnis; however, they were forced to

Future

munities. In
idge over the
nd provide a

te 66
d crosses
Route 66,
nerica's
During their
nsported

The Rise and Fall of Times Beach

Times Beach got its name from the St. Louis Times newspaper and from the beach along the Meramec River where the town was established. In 1926, the same year Route 66 became a federal highway, the St. Louis Times newspaper sold land lots in the resort area of Times Beach to the public for $67.50 with the purchase of a six-month subscription to its paper. The town never quite blossomed into the summer retreat the newspaper advertised that it would become. Instead, it turned into a small, middle-class town of roughly 2,000 people.

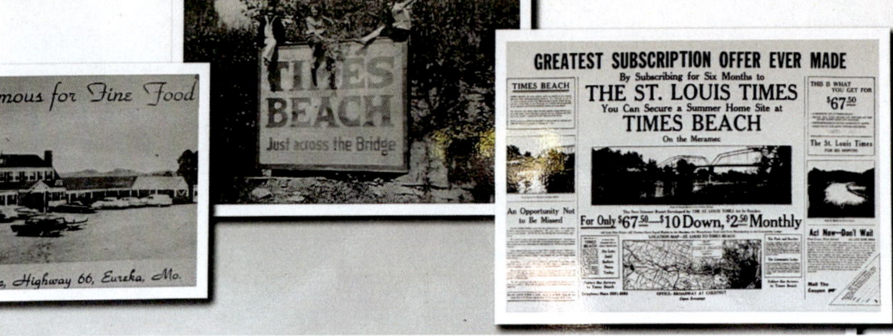

CHANGING TIMES At the Route 66 State Park near Eureka, Missouri, nothing remains of Times Beach—once a thriving resort community, later an EPA Superfund dioxin cleanup site—except an interpretive placard at the old bridge overlook. We read the exhibit as a cautionary tale of what *not* to do as a newspaper promotion...

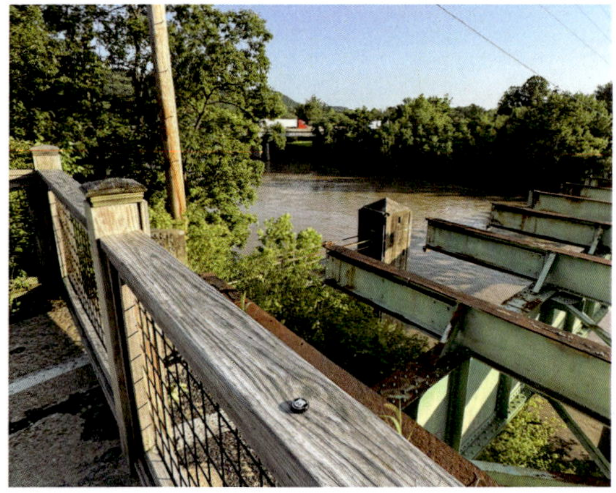

ROAD TO NOWHERE Today the decking of the Route 66 bridge has been removed, and most of the traffic passing by on the parallel stretch of Interstate have no clue to the region's rich Route 66 history.

leave most of their possessions behind, including a camera. The *Joplin Globe* developed and printed the film, which showed now-legendary photos of Bonnie holding Clyde at mock gunpoint, and of Bonnie with her foot on a car fender, posed with a pistol in her hand and cigar in her mouth."

Yes, we rubbernecked at the modest 34th Street home that was briefly the gangsters' hideout. But more of interest to us was the city's twenty-first-century story.

Our generation recalls Joplin as victim of a mile-wide EF5 tornado strike in May 2011. A 10x20 mural, "On the Wings of Butterflies," stands today on the site of a hospital destroyed in that storm. Artist Eric Haun painted another mural, titled "161," that features one butterfly for each of those who perished in the massive event. A "butterfly effect" hatched other representations now incorporated into artworks around the city.

"Going forward from the tornado," wrote Joplin Convention & Visitors Bureau director Patrick Tuttle in a Four States Homepage article a decade after the disaster, "Joplin is not defined by the one event, but instead as a town they must focus on recovery and look forward—which the town has done over the past 10 years, and the murals represent that."

Kay and I spent a delightful afternoon chasing butterflies—and other brilliantly rendered images—all around the city.

At last, determining belatedly that we'd benefit from a printed guide, we stopped in at the Convention & Visitor Bureau, located in the elegant former Newman's Department Store on Main Street, now its city hall.

Tourism assistant Donna Miller plied us with helpful brochures and maps. We happily purchased lightweight souvenirs, these days in the form of ubiquitous, colorful die-cut stickers smaller than the bumper promos of yore. They travel well, go in the mail to friends back home, and fit easily into journals or on guitar cases or bulletin boards.

Noting the poster reproduction framed in the building's foyer, I (an art student in earlier days) remarked how much I admired the Thomas Hart Benton work it incorporated. Missourian Benton's ruralist style had long captivated me, and I recalled for Miller how powerfully the energetic composition of his 1928 painting "Boomtown" portrayed the Borger oil-boom community back in our home state of Texas.

"Oh, come with me!" Miller exclaimed in excitement, practically dragging me by the arm out the office doorway and around the corner.

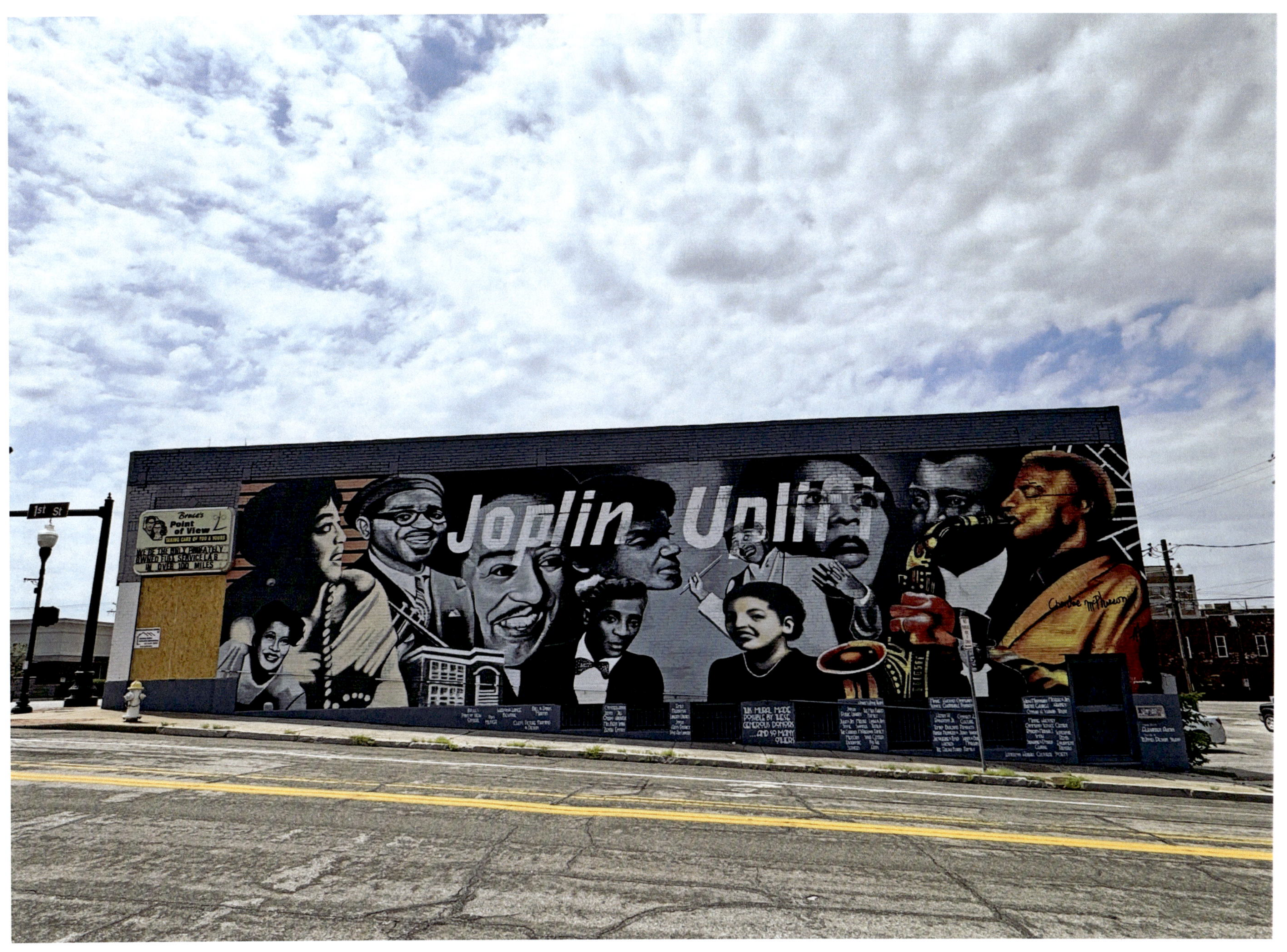

"JOPLIN UPLIFT" The mural by Kansas City artist Alexander Austin at 102 S. Main Street on the north side of Bruce's Point of View Optical celebrates Joplin's rich Black history, including the historic Joplin Uplift newspaper.

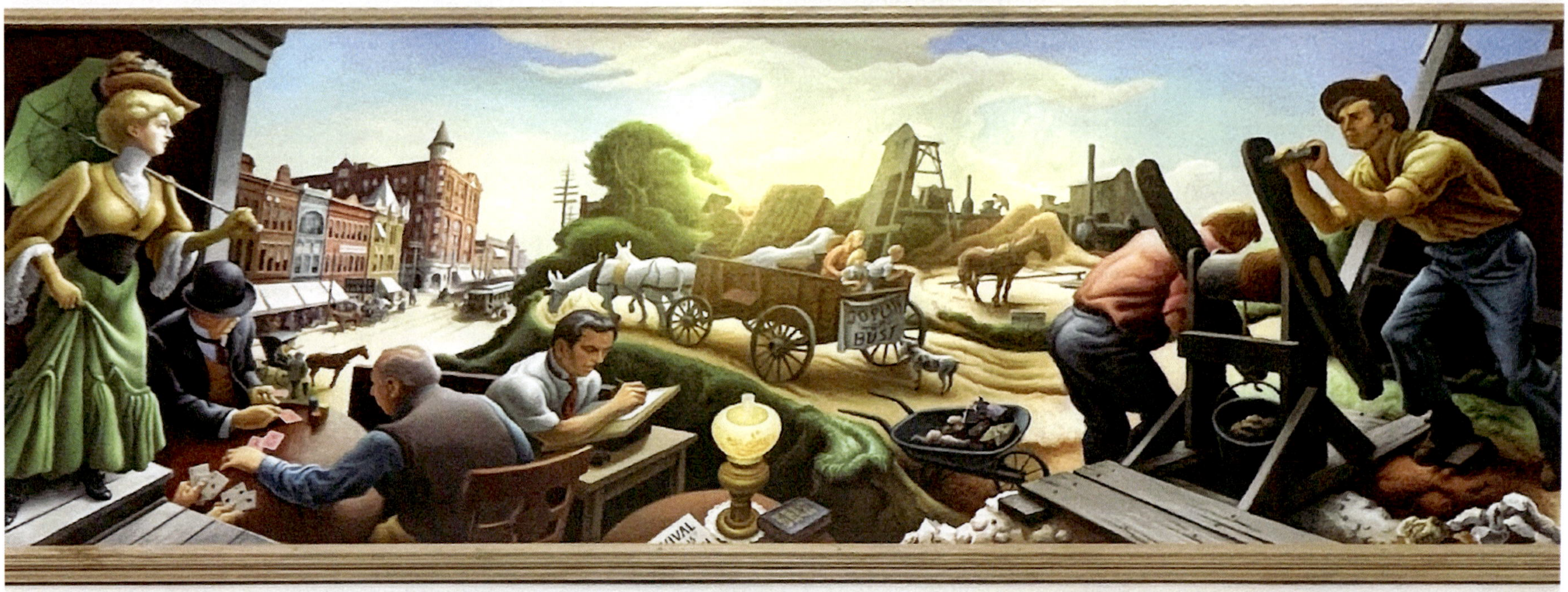

There, stretched out above the entry, was Benton's *original*.

"Joplin at the Turn of the Century, 1896–1906," we learned, is Benton's only autobiographical work. (Yes, we spotted his younger likeness—above, in the red necktie—sketching among the milling throngs in his composition.) Dedicated in 1973 to honor Joplin's 100th birthday, this mural was the last piece Benton signed before his death in 1975.

City Hall also displays an exhibition on how their showpiece came about, and continuing the tradition, the 2010 mural "Route 66, Joplin, Missouri"—by Benton's grandson Anthony Benton Gude—also graces its walls. The building is open to the public Monday through Friday, 8 a.m. to 5 p.m., and by appointment on weekends.

You showed us, Missouri: you showed us a great time. Thank you. ☞

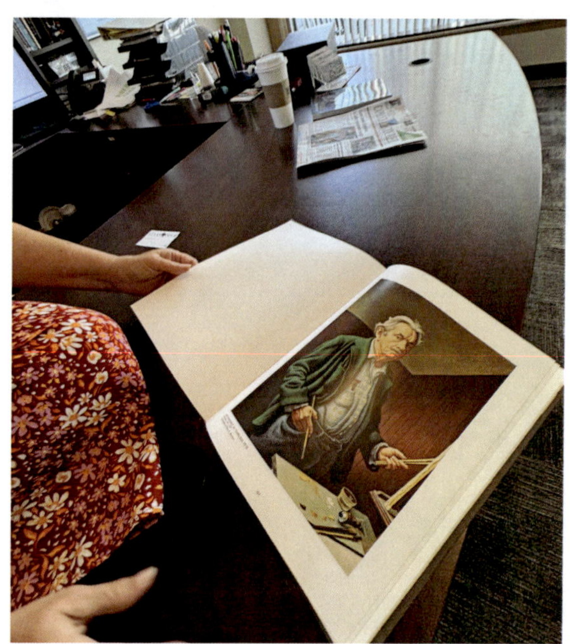

PAINTER THOMAS HART BENTON completed a mural commission for Joplin's Centennial in 1973 (above), and the city's Convention & Visitor Bureau keeps a wealth of reference information on hand (right).

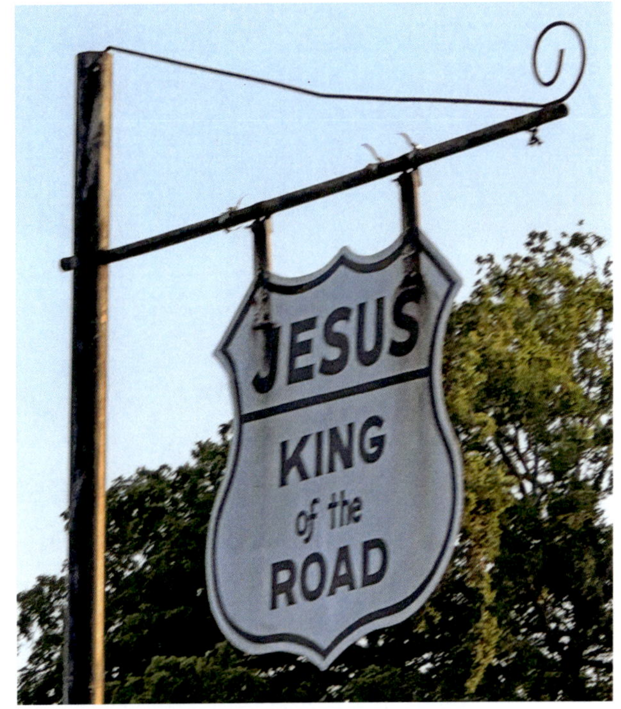

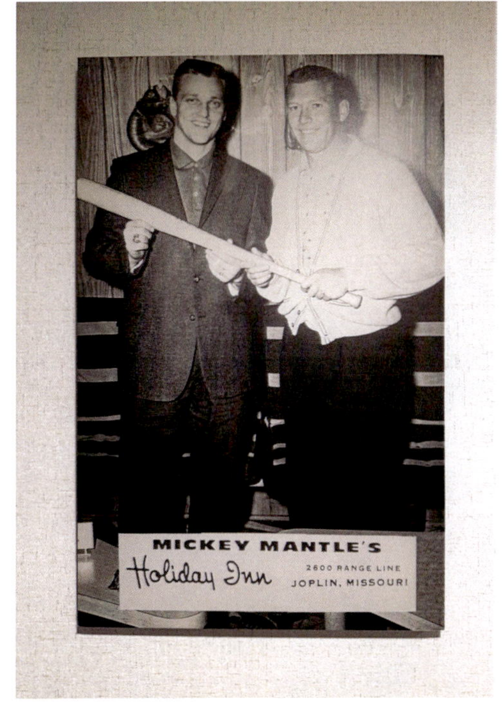

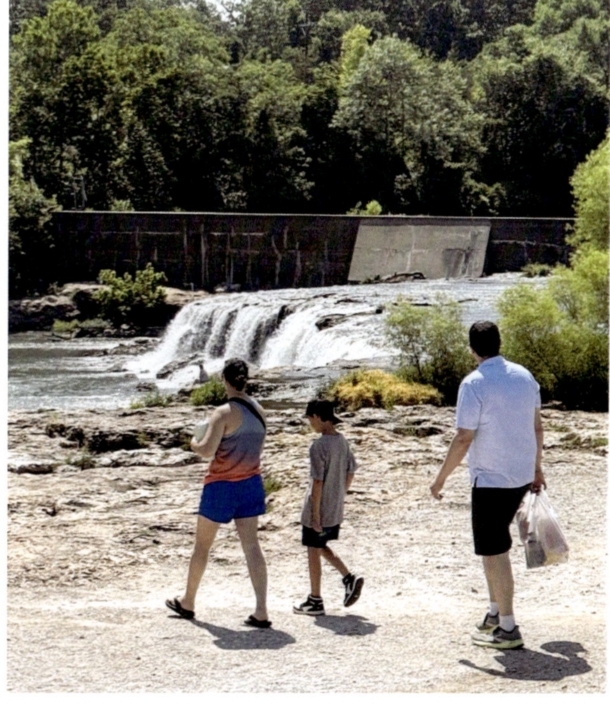

GRAND FALLS just outside of Joplin is the largest continuously running waterfall in a state crisscrossed by rivers—at 12 feet high.

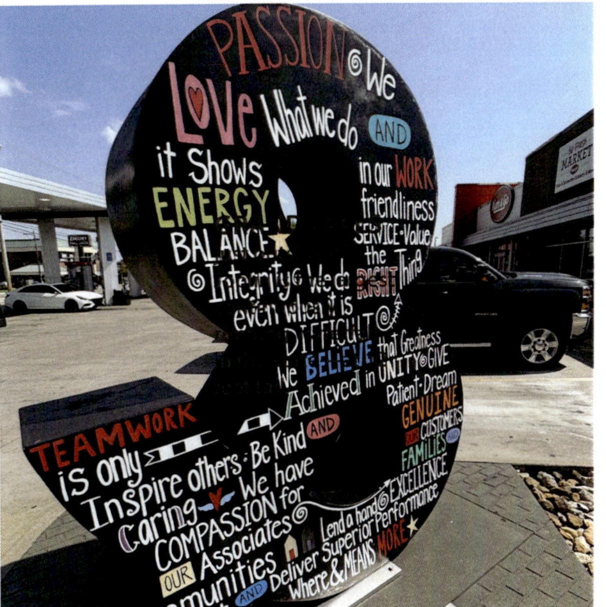

MOVE OVER, ROGER MILLER in Cuba, Missouri (because Jesus is, after all, my rock, my sword AND my shield, in the book of Randy Travis).

CARRYING THE MANTLE for the Holiday Inn Brand, the famous slugger Mickey Mantle, a native of Oklahoma, invested in a Joplin hotel property in 1957; he promoted it as the 200th Holiday Inn, displaying memorabilia from his baseball career. Our lodging for the night was the city's newest in the chain, which displays memorabilia from the earlier hotel.

AND . . . a sculptural ampersand at the Kum & Go convenience store, 3434 S. Rangeline Road in Joplin, celebrates the company slogan "Where & Means More." (Readers take note: Since our 2024 Route 66 through-drive, the chain has sold to a competitor. Does the art remain? We'll find out next trip!)

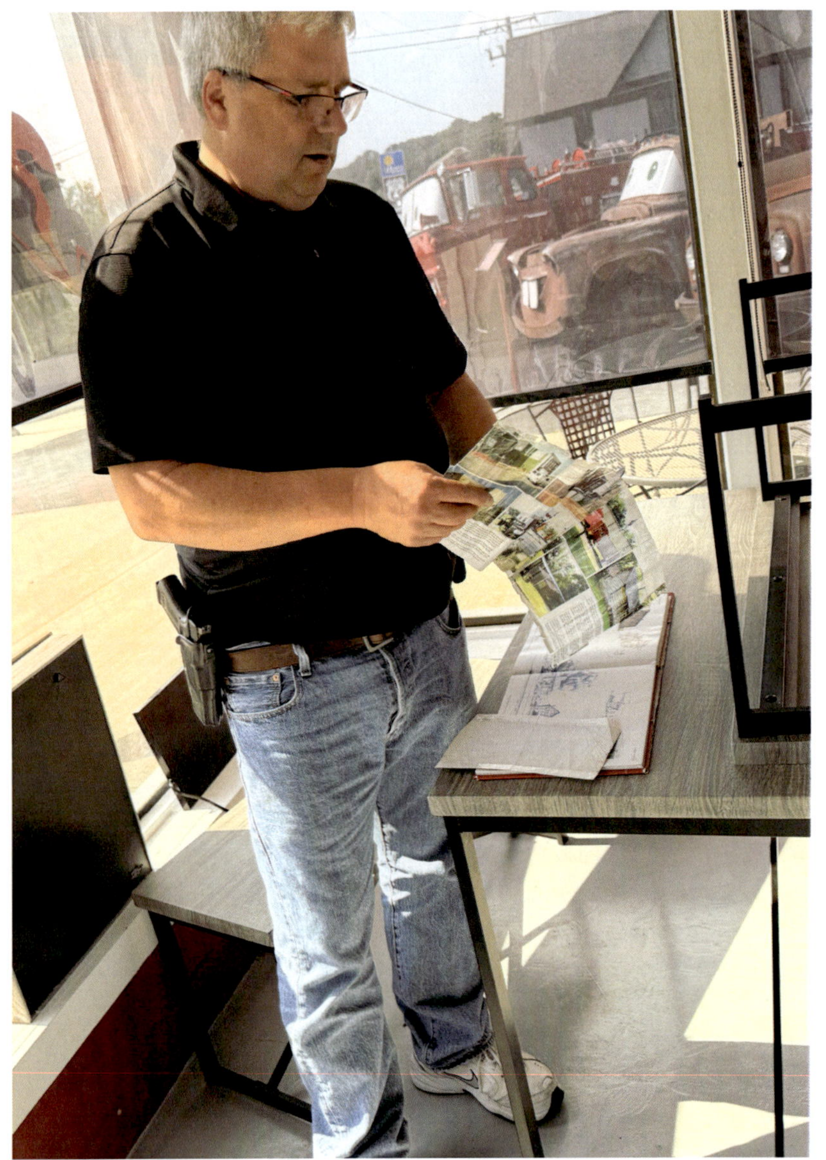

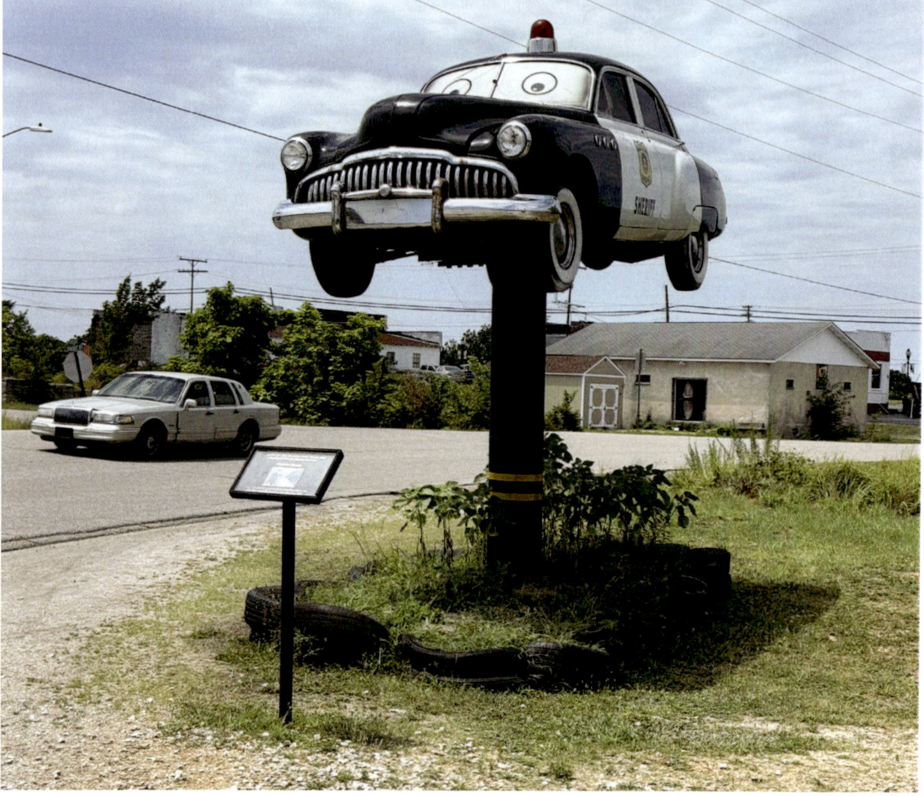

A REPLICA SHERIFF'S CRUISER reminds visitors to slow down as they enter Galena, Kansas. I couldn't help hearing in my head the gravelly voice of that *Cars* character, provided by longtime Route 66 champion Michael Wallis of Tulsa.

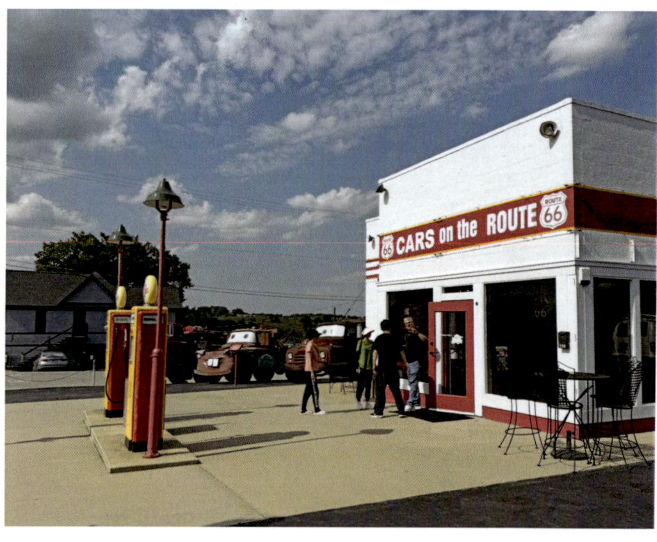

CARS ON THE ROUTE is the updated name of roadie Renee Charles's souvenir shop (right) in Galena, Kansas, which encapsulates the automobile culture of the Mother Road but also the pop-culture phenomenon of the 2006 Disney/Pixar *Cars* animated film. Her husband, police chief Billy Joe Charles showed us his scrapbooks from the research and filming that began in 2001. Chief Charles retired from his post only a few weeks after our delightful meetup with him, but we hope we didn't prompt his decision.

CHAPTER THREE

Not in Kansas anymore? Think again

OF THE EIGHT STATES through which Route 66 once passed—and its historic remnants still do—Kansas claims the least, by far. But that 13.2-mile-long elbow jutting into the state's southeasternmost corner has played an outsized role in the culture of the Mother Road, and in its survival for enthusiasts to drive today.

In the second half of the twentieth century, progress in the form of one of the U.S.'s earliest high-speed Interstate highways—I-44, which extends now from St. Louis to Wichita Falls, Texas—replaced Route 66 along a wider and straighter path.

(Roadgeek trivia, per Wikipedia: As US 66 was being bypassed by Interstate 44, the Route 66 Association requested the designation "Interstate 66" for I-44 from St. Louis to Oklahoma City; transportation officials rejected the request.)

Part of that straighter-path philosophy was to eliminate Route 66's right-angle into Kansas entirely.

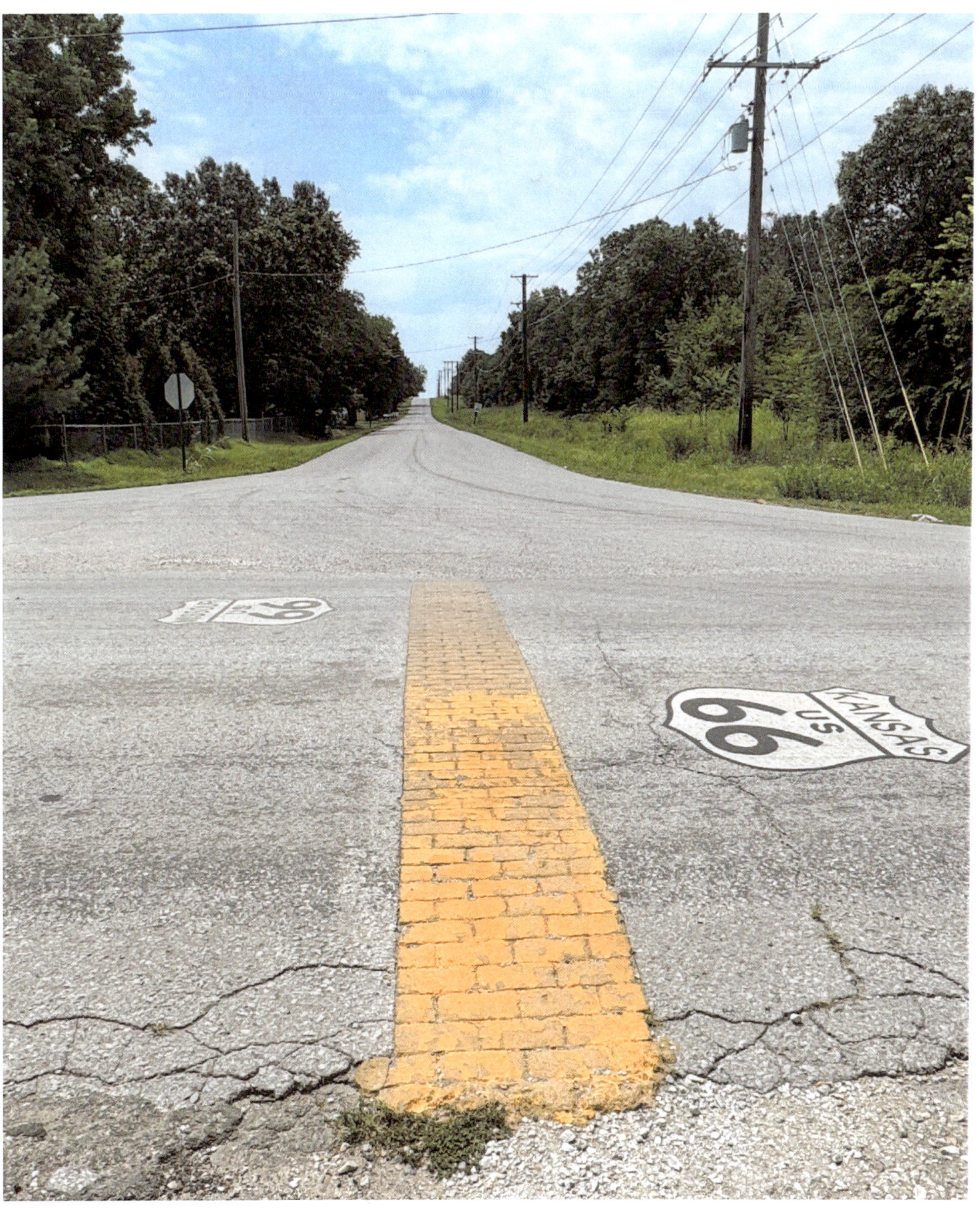

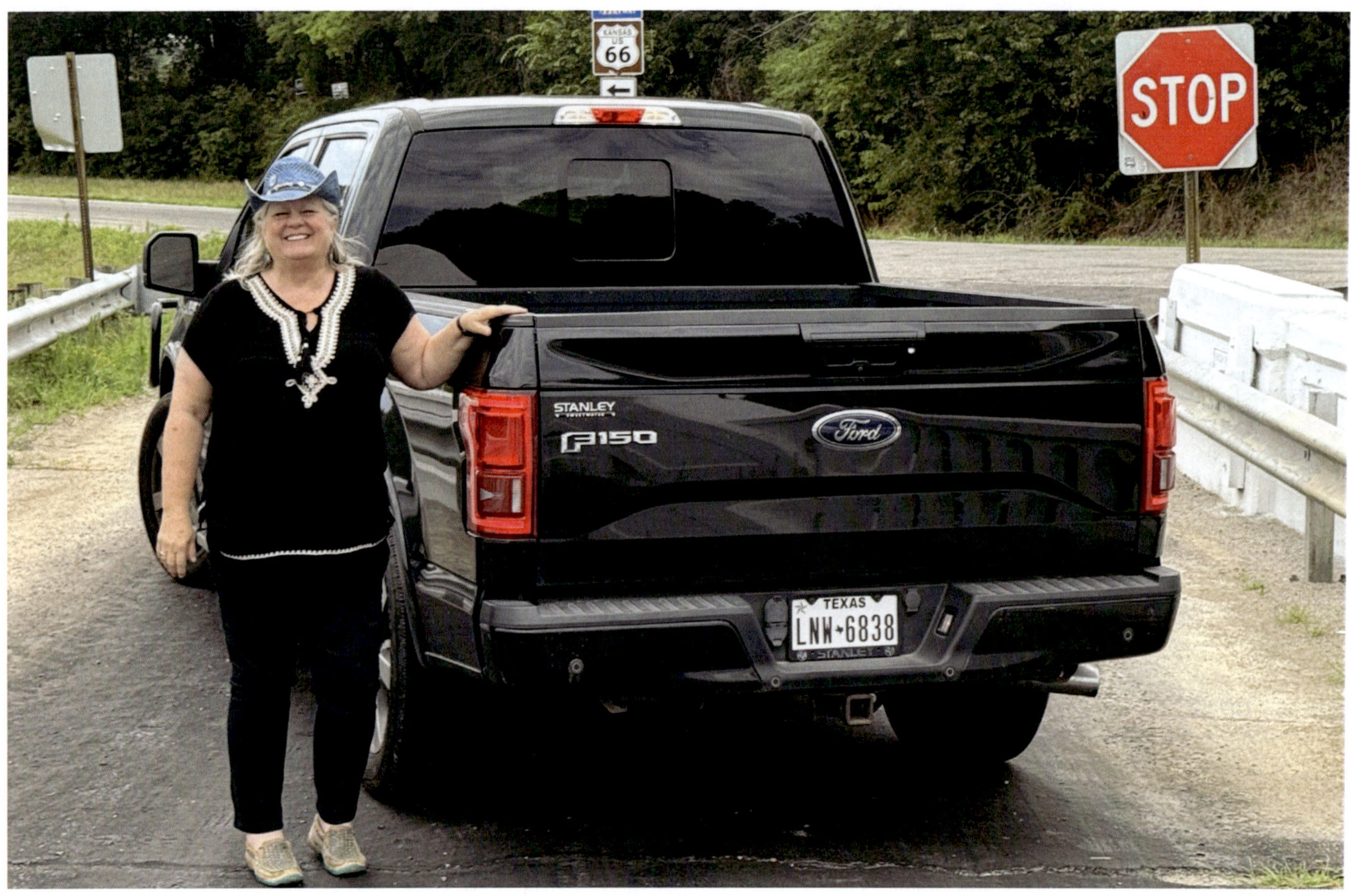

RAINBOW BRIDGE In Riverton, Kansas, the Marsh Arch bridge over Brush Creek is the only surviving bridge of this type on the entire length of Route 66.

As we departed Missouri and crossed the yellow-brick stripe on old 66 that marks the state line into Kansas, we at first wondered why anyone might care. Then, around the bend, a delightful mishmash of Route 66 reminders hove into view.

A drive-through aluminum highway shield.

A pole design pointing to destinations as disparate as Amarillo, TX (474 miles), Tucumcari, NM (579), and Santa Monica Pier, CA (with miles left blank, but it'll take us another week to get there so we know it's a lot).

And spying from atop an iron post just as sneakily as he might've done behind a billboard in the 2006 *Cars* movie, a twin of the Sheriff's 1949 black-and-white-with-cherry-on-top police cruiser.

We laughed when we also discovered a facsimile of Luigi the Fiat peeking out of a garage door.

Turns out we'd barely scratched the surface.

Back in 2001, Galena, Kansas, provided a pivotal bit of pop culture during Pixar director John Lasseter's scouting expedition for an animated film he'd begun to envision during a cross-country family vacation the summer before.

There, outside a run-down Kan-O-Tex filling station, his team spotted a rusted, run-down vintage tow truck. And he met the truck's owner, who possessed the redoubtable skill of bending his double-jointed legs in opposite directions.

Kay and I, knowing only a few tidbits of this history, cruised right on

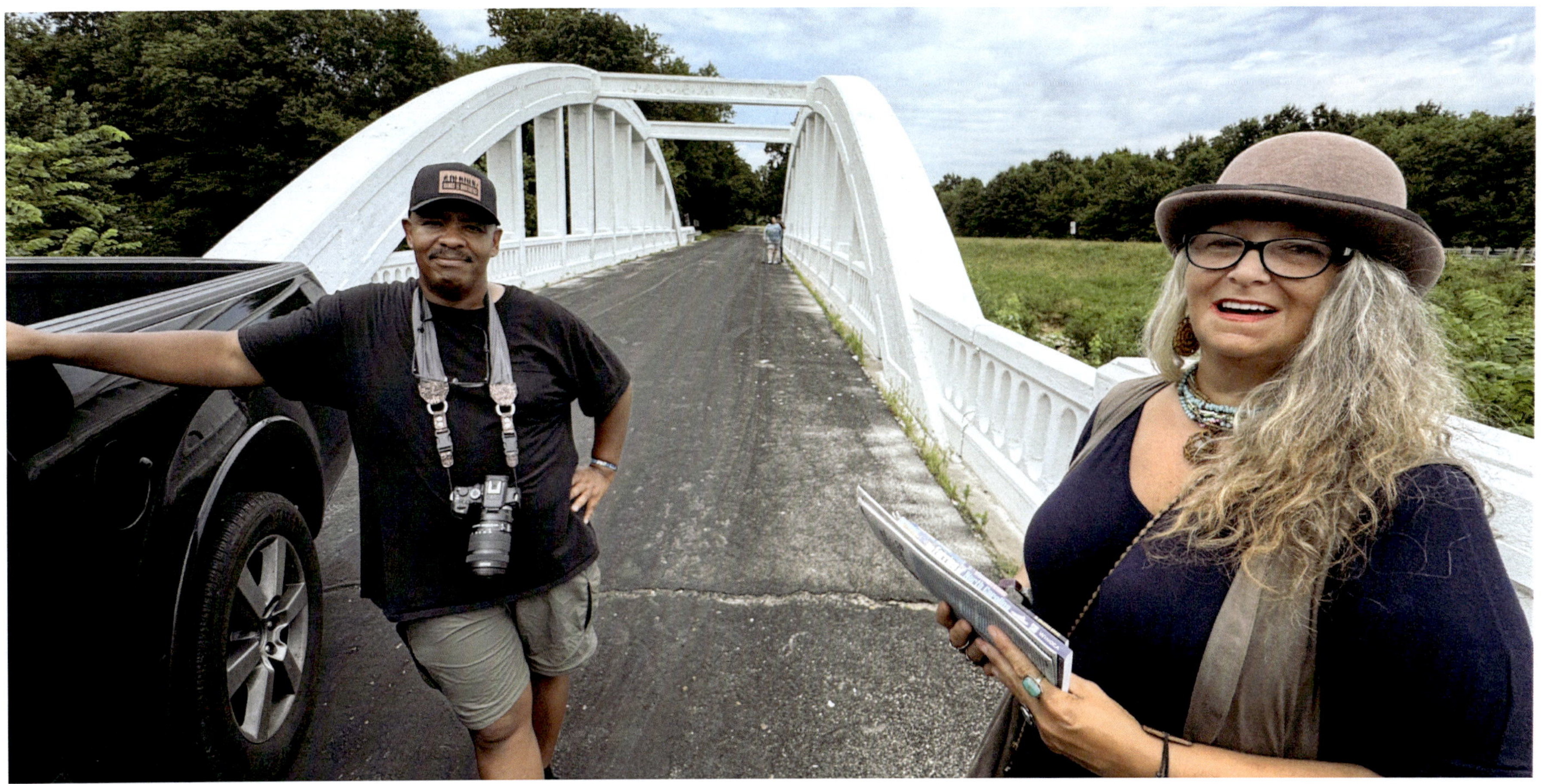

through Galena, most of whose establishments weren't yet open for the day. Right up the road in Baxter Springs was Kansas' Route 66 Visitor Center. The restored Phillips 66 station also offered public restrooms. This building *did* have its lights on and welcome sign out.

I swung open the door into the tiny lobby. Before either of us could inquire directions to the loo, the greeter bellowed out, "What's your favorite character in *Cars*?"

"Um … Sally the Porsche?" I ventured, in solidarity with my sex.

"Wrong."

I tried again, the correct answer dawning on me after taking in the memorabilia and photos that festooned every corner of the station's walls.

"Mater!" I supplied, slapping my forehead.

Dean "Crazy-Legs" Walker proceeded to perform for us the famous stunt that had inspired the *Cars* team to endow their lovable tow truck with its unforgettable reverse-gear quirk.

Walker's only one of the legendary personalities who lent their true stories and knowledge to the movie—which in turn brought multiple generations of new fans to experience the real Mother Road for themselves.

AT THE 1923 'RAINBOW' MARSH ARCH BRIDGE in Riverton, Kansas, photographers Rick Pulley (above left) and Tammy Roberts took advantage of the scenic spot for some publicity takes. Pulley, also a musician, supports a veterans project called Band of Brothers.

Back up the road in Galena, once a run-down, rusted-out mining town bypassed by the big-muscle Interstate, authenticity fed the inspiration for a pop-culture phenomenon that would eventually drive dollars back into tiny-town economies for 2,448 miles.

The Kansas towns Kay and I visited multiple times that day—motoring back and forth into Missouri and across to Oklahoma to photograph the Route in differing lights—epitomized the evolution of a road from Roaring '20s enthusiasm to '50s heyday to crumbling '80s ruin and back again.

We thrilled at the chance to drive the one remaining segment of a Marsh Arch "rainbow" bridge, across Brush Creek between Riverton and Baxter Springs, which launched us into fond memories of crossing a similarly preserved example last year in the *Home Town Takeover* town of Fort Morgan, Colorado.

We gleaned even more appreciation for these sites from the streaming audio content we'd discovered at the outset of our journey, Anthony Arno's *Route 66 Podcast.* Educator Arno's format includes bits of backstory, but the companionable host mostly provides generous stretches of airtime for his interview guests to ramble at will. It's an informative and inspiring way to become acquainted with the many children of the Mother Road.

We'd already listened to the wonderful opening segment with Michael Wallis, author of *Route 66: The Mother Road* (first published in 1990 and updated since then) and voice of the Sheriff in *Cars.*

We finished our afternoon in Kansas learning from a few more of the road's characters, warriors and champions. A lovely golden light settled over the old Kan-O-Tex Station, where a visiting family snapped photos and waved good-bye to the real-life local police chief, who's married to the station's co-owner and was making a few fixups to the place. We marveled at the ripple effect that's brought Route 66 nostalgia to a whole new generation.

That's a heck of a lot of value for just 13.2 miles. ☞

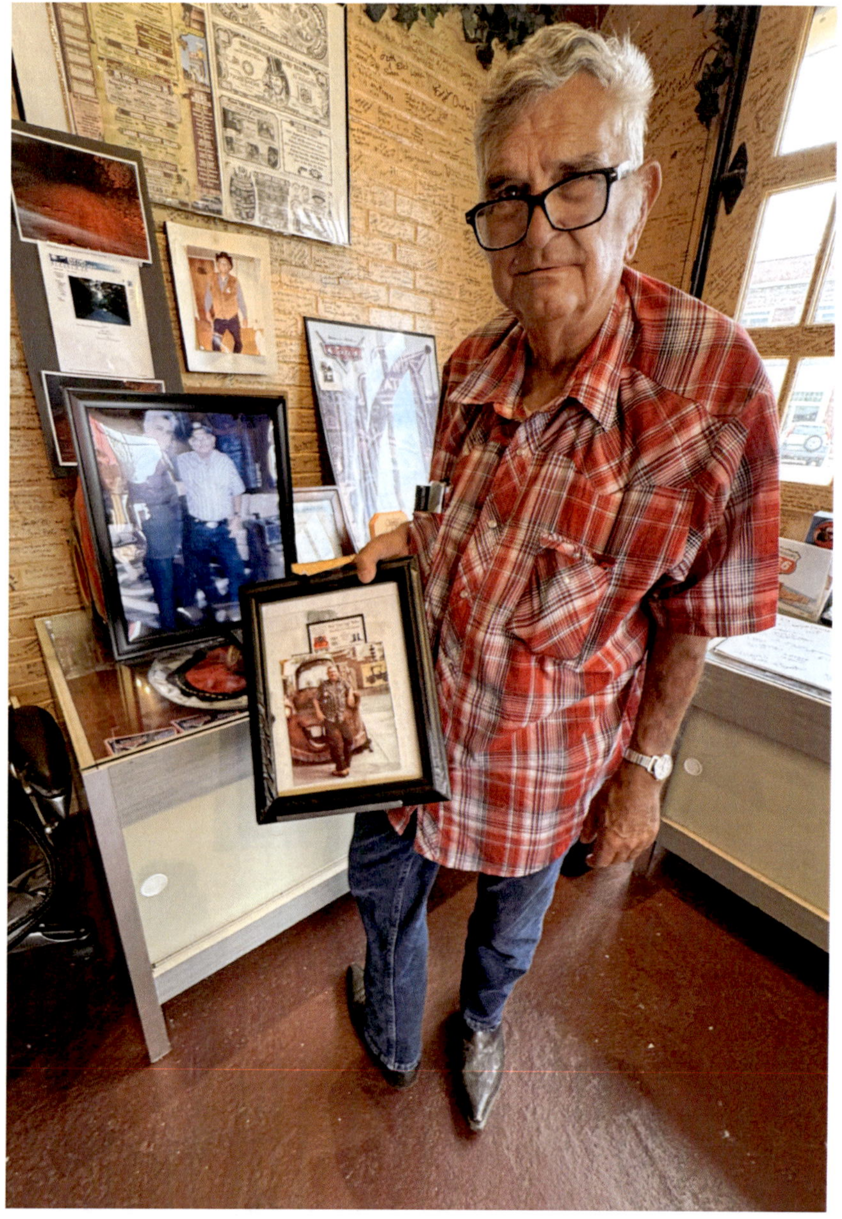

DOUBLE-JOINTED JOINT At the Baxter Springs visitor center Dean "Crazy-Legs" Walker demonstrated the stunt that had inspired the *Cars* team's lovable tow truck. Nicknamed for his ability to turn his legs backward, Walker had received a lifetime achievement award from the Kansas Historic Route 66 Association a few weeks before our surprise visit.

READ MORE about the real-life inspirations for the Disney/Pixar *Cars* characters in a piece by Amarillo author Nick Gerlich in *Route* Magazine, www.routemagazine.us/stories/the-cars-story

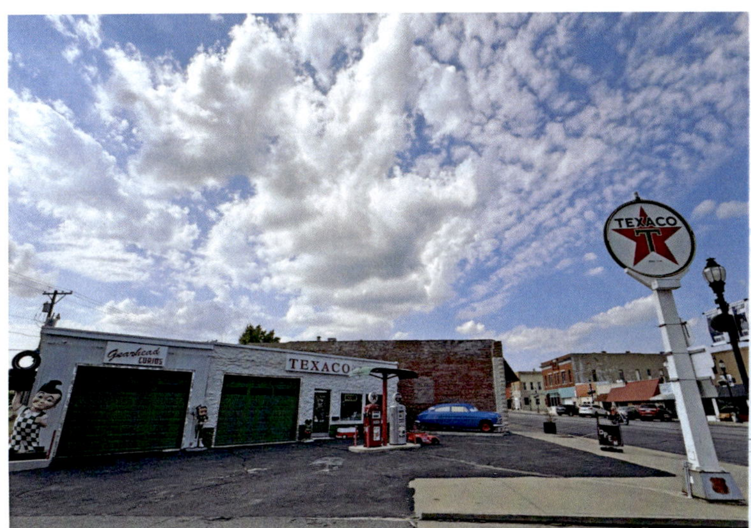

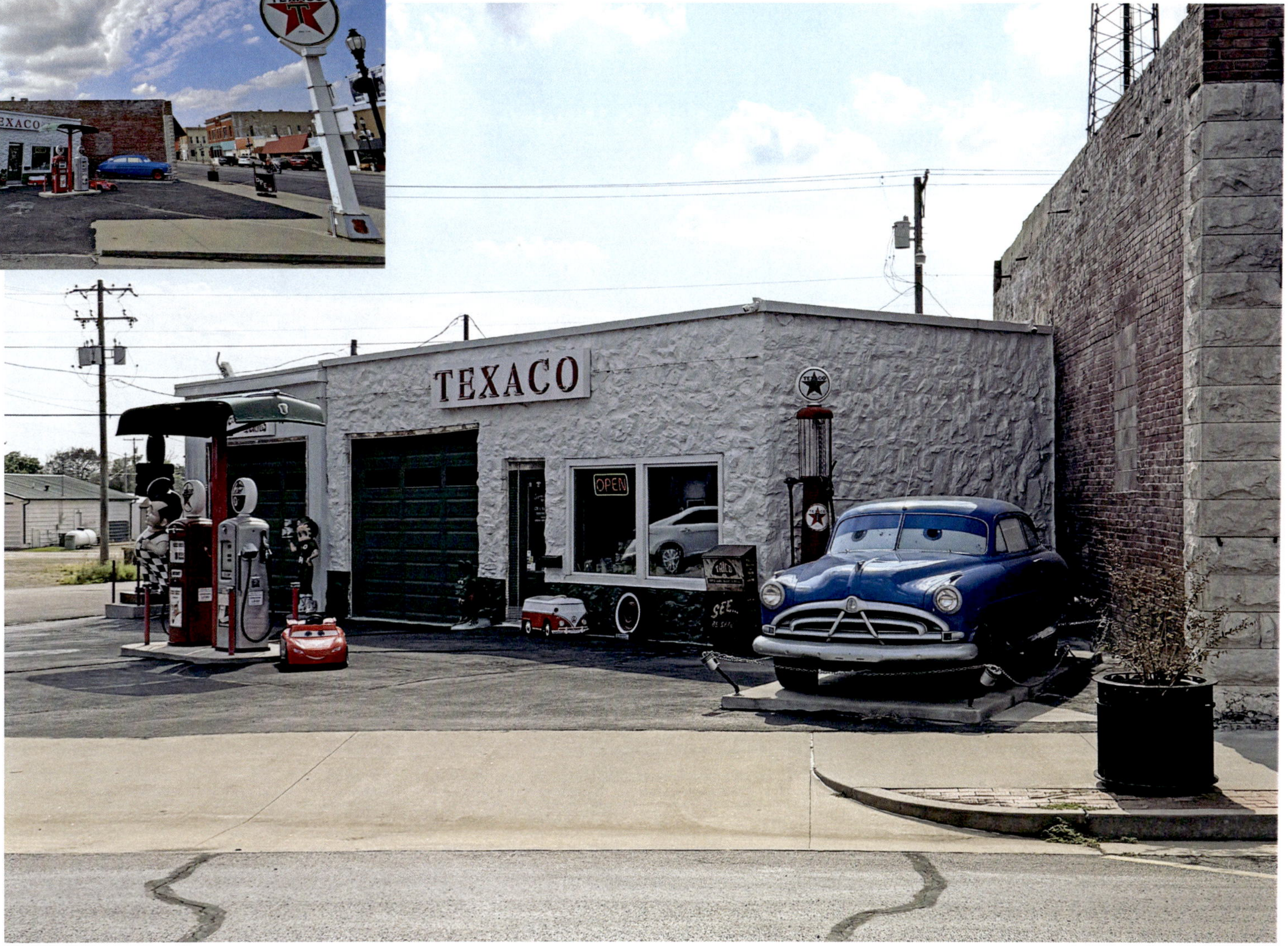

IN THE SECOND HALF of the twentieth century, "progress" replaced Route 66 along a wider and straighter path. Part of that straighter-path philosophy, in 1961, was to eliminate Route 66's right-angle into Kansas entirely. But in 20026 it was the idiosyncratic inhabitants of the state's 12.8 (some say 13.2, depending on how you measure it) old Route 66 miles that helped revive The Mother Road—via one game-changing animated film.

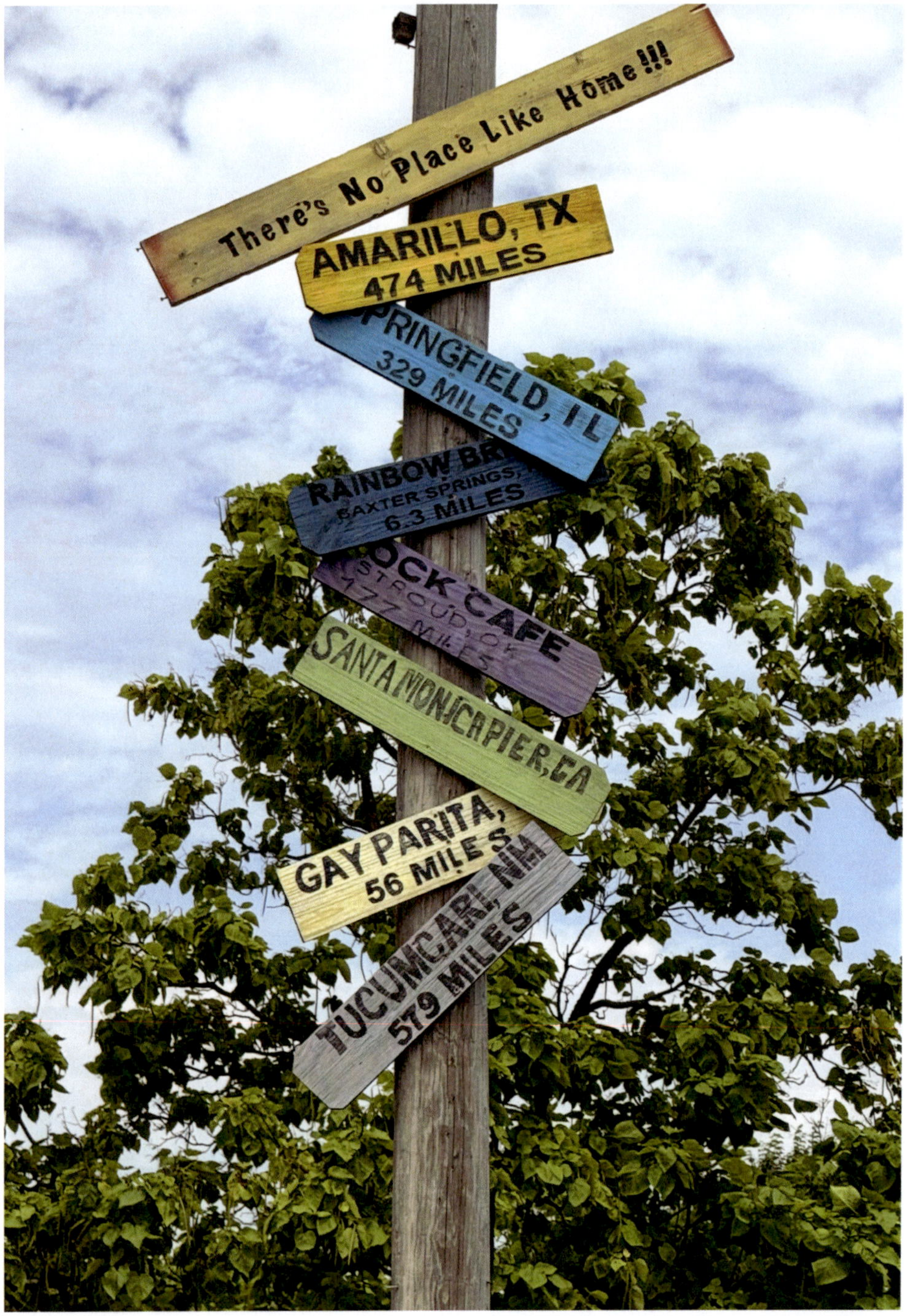

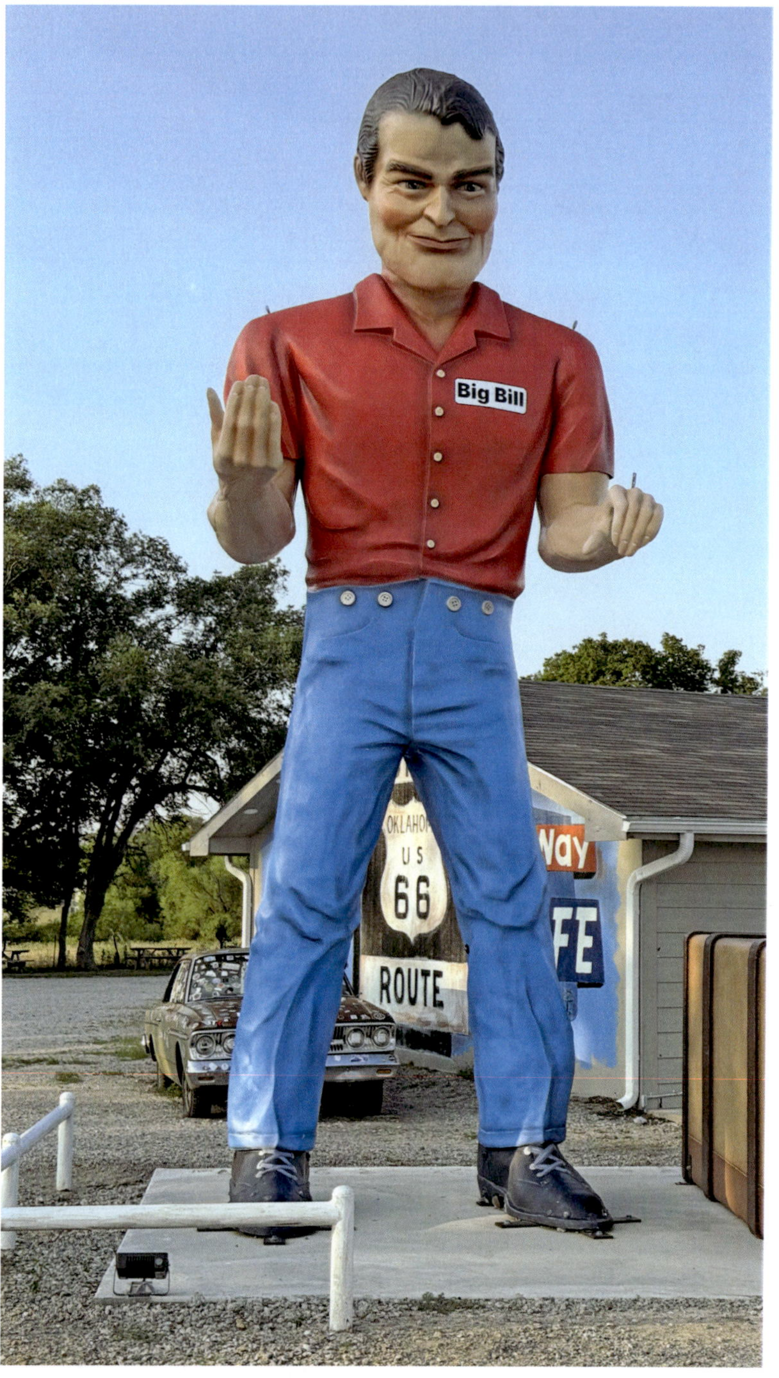

There's No Place Like Home!!!
AMARILLO, TX
474 MILES
SPRINGFIELD, IL
329 MILES
RAINBOW BR
BAXTER SPRINGS,
6.3 MILES
OCK CAFE
STROUD, OK
177 MILES
SANTA MONICA PIER, CA
GAY PARITA,
56 MILES
TUCUMCARI, NM
579 MILES
Big Bill
OKLAHOMA
US
66
ROUTE
way
FE

"BRING IT ON," 21-foot-tall Big Bill of Vinita, Oklahoma, seems to say, or maybe just "Welcome to Oklahoma." Relocated to the town of 5,500 a few years earlier to help draw vehicle traffic off the turnpike and into Beth Hilburn's Hi-Way Cafe on Route 66, the fiberglass figure was given his current name in memory of the proprietor's late father. By the time we'd reached Oklahoma, spotting Muffler Men and Uniroyal Gals had become a frequent, but always-delightful surprise, and we were grateful to have learned their backstory so early in the trip at the American Giants Museum—though by now Illinois itself seemed a distant memory. The signpost at far left, in Galena, Kansas, beckoned us to famous landmarks in Oklahoma and beyond, like Stroud's Rock Café—and the Santa Monica Pier, apparently too distant a mileage to calculate.

CHAPTER FOUR

Oklahoma, green hills to Panhandle

OKLAHOMA HAS MORE DRIVABLE MILES of Route 66 than any other state. And "drivable," as twenty-first-century roadies know, is all-important.

I digress for a moment here, from Oklahoma's varied and fascinating tourist attractions—and its music legends from Woody Guthrie to Reba McEntire to Garth Brooks—to consider that notion of "drivable."

You wouldn't, in the year 2024, necessarily attempt to motor west over every crumbling vestige of circa-1926 pavement that still exists. Or would you? Some purists consider such an itinerary the holy grail, as Appalachian Trail through-hikers insist on walking the continuous footpath from Georgia to Maine (or vice versa) without cheating by hitching a ride during severe weather, or bypassing steep passages too challenging for your physique, or yielding to the constraints of real-world career or family.

As a dedicated roadgeek myself, I know from previous tries at all of the 1916 Bankhead Highway from one end of Texas to the other, or US 83 ("The Last American Highway") from Mexico to Canada, or even the 2,554 high-speed miles of I-40, that this isn't always practical or even possible.

An early thoroughfare that might've promised a continuous route from end to end simply doesn't exist along every mile once the vagaries of climate and bureaucracy have taken their toll. Alignments stretch or straighten; stronger bridges are built; signs come and go. Departments of transportation draft new maps, and old designations disappear.

Here in Oklahoma, that's abundantly true. Any attempt to stick to the Mother Road across her 432 miles made famous by the Okie Joads of *The*

Grapes of Wrath will meet with frustration at numerous diversions onto city streets, toll roads, or that blandest of east-west Interstates, the 40. The Ross/McClanahan "Here It Is" maps (mentioned in a previous chapter) are your best shot. Even then, flooding and deteriorating pavement might frustrate your aims, as another author of our audiobook entertainment, Rick Antonson, once experienced in a very wet Sooner State.

For Kay and me, in mid-July 2024, flooding wasn't a problem. It hadn't rained a drop since the deluge in Atlanta, Illinois. So our first challenge, in Ottawa County, Oklahoma, was to locate the storied Ribbon Road.

The highway anomaly—a stretch of vintage pavement only 9 feet wide that had existed for a decade before being swept up in Route 66—was under siege that very week. We'd read in the papers about the Miami (Oklahoma) city council's threat to grind up the relict of badly deteriorated concrete-and-asphalt sandwich the road had become. It's understandable that no planer or miller could scrape that pavement without damaging road and equipment alike. And the result would be only a worse grosgrain-ribbon texture than exists at present, which holds any automobile's horses to about 10 miles per hour.

I'd signed the online petition to forestall the council's action. I reached out to Oklahoma 66's head honcho, Rhys Martin of Tulsa, with whom I'd crossed paths in earlier preservation initiatives.

Oh, and I wrote a song, of course. Stay tuned (page 65 if you're curious).

> *Our first challenge, in Ottawa County, Oklahoma, was to locate the legendary Ribbon Road.*

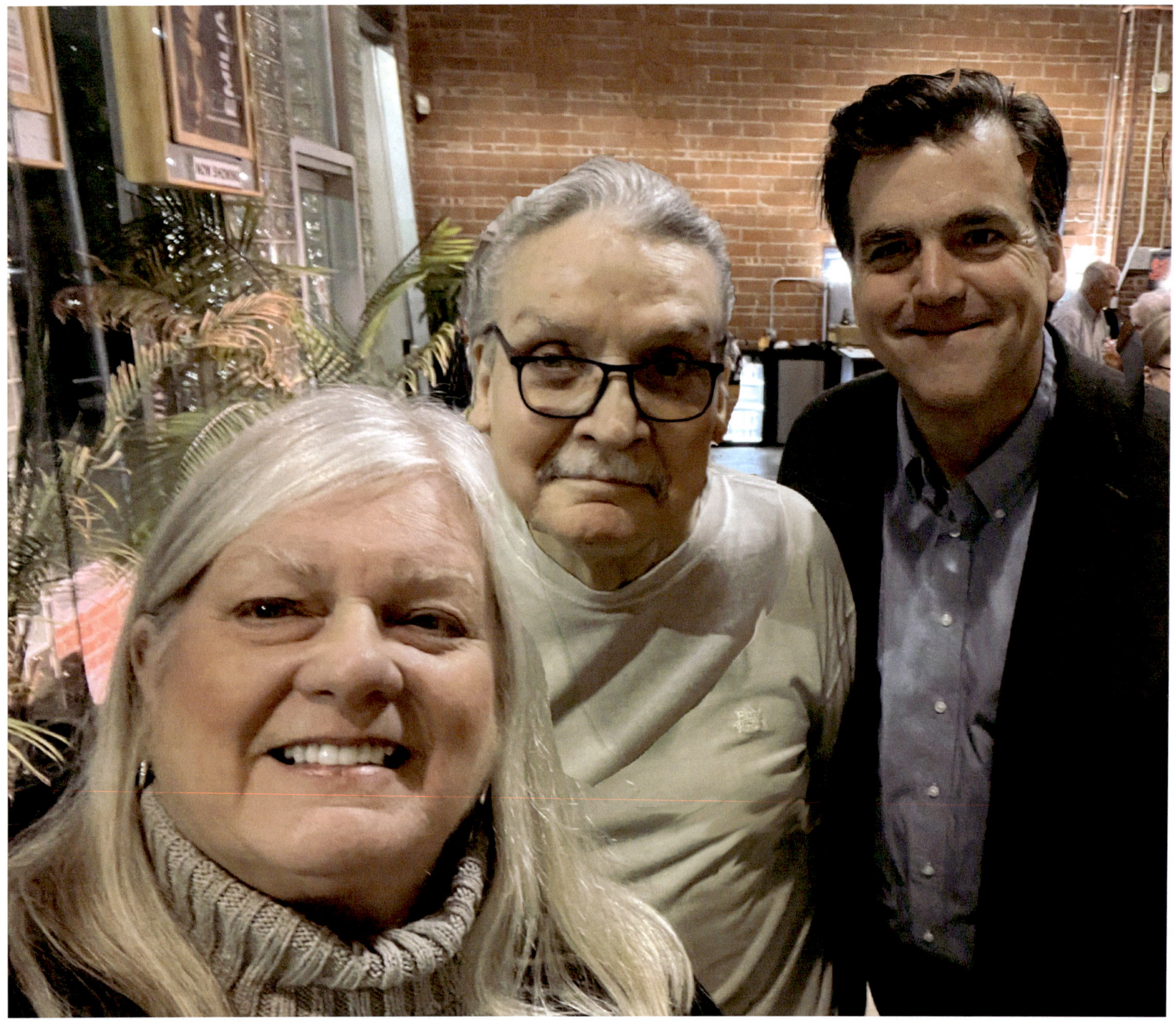

AMERICAN ODYSSEY Tulsa's vibrant arts and outdoor scene has beckoned us back from Texas repeatedly. On a return for Kay's birthday a few months after our summer 2024 through-drive, we had the delight of meeting Route champions Michael Wallis (center) and John Paget (right), who screened Paget's original film collaboration *Route 66: An American Odyssey* in advance of a planned 2026 remake as *The Main Street of America*. "There are lots of straight roads," Wallis advised the audience. "You need to stick to the *crooked* roads."

Following directions provided by numerous websites (the Historical Marker Database is one of the best), we set out from Miami southwest toward E 140 Road. At a 90-degree elbow amid field and forest, we knew we'd found it: that 9-foot-wide roadway edged by concrete curbing, recognizable from many photos.

It could only be the unique-on-66 Sidewalk Highway, supposedly designed by a 1912 highway department too strapped for cash to complete a full 18-foot two-lane road. The same budget dollars allocated to a single lane could stretch twice the miles, they reasoned.

Originally part of the Ozark Trail, a regional auto route that predated the national Route 66, the Ribbon Road has become a treasured artifact. To replace its deteriorated surface with modern material and safety marking, partisans argue, would be akin to rebuilding the Parthenon out of PVC. But few preservation remedies remain, except to leave it as is—to further crackle and pop and weather away to dust.

We advance reverently, the setting sun drifting occasionally through the sentry rows of boxelder and blackjack, trying to prevent our Firestones from inflicting further damage. No other vehicle passes to force us onto the narrow shoulder. By the time we reach the marble marker at the "preserved" curve most travelers manage to find just off today's US 59, we're quiet, somber. If it's true, as poet Frost wrote, that nothing gold can stay, is asphalt destined always for a similar fate?

"Completed in 1922 as Federal Highway Project No. 8. Running 15.46 miles from Miami to Afton," it reads. "The only remaining 9′ section of original pavement on the old Route 66 system, taken out of service in 1937. A National Register of Historic Places Site."

Whatever of Old 66 lies ahead of us in Oklahoma, we expect it will pale in comparison to this most elegiac of road relics.

Over the next 24 hours our rambles will take us into Tulsa past Big Bill the Muffler Man at Vinita, over the Pryor Creek iron bridge at Chelsea, past the Will Rogers Museum at Claremore and on to the delightful Blue Whale at Catoosa. As we stop for all of these it becomes apparent that Oklahoma will require a return trip, for we haven't even reached its midsection of Route 66 riches.

Time's wingèd chariot presses on, and after our in-depth tour of Tulsa's Church Studio (where rock-piano legend and native son Leon Russell

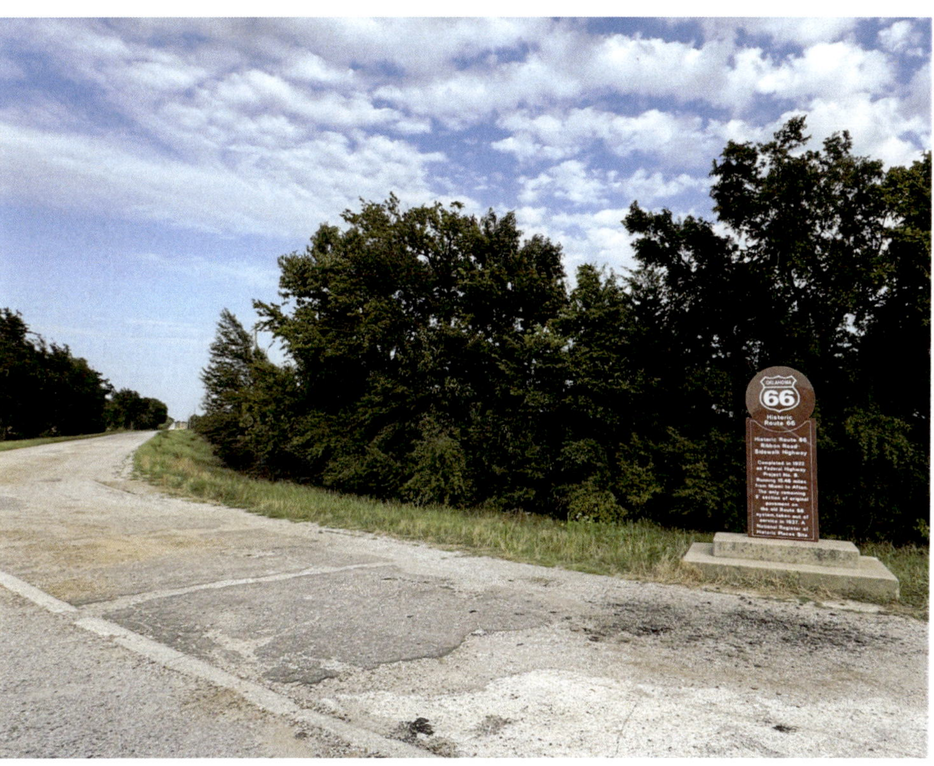

THE RIBBON ROAD outside Miami, Oklahoma, is a remnant of the solitary stretch of Route 66 that was built in 1912 (before the Route was officially designated) as a single lane. Compare the even worse condition of the road in our 2024 photo with the slightly earlier one on the Ribbon Road website, https://oklahomaroute66.com/ribbon

transformed a former house of worship into a world-class recording studio, still a vital force today) the inexorable river of I-40 sweeps us along through the capital city and westward across rivers and plains. Night falls on us at last at Weatherford, having passed our last hours of twilight traversing the two-lane roller-coaster of what Google Maps calls "U.S. Bicycle Route 66" past Bridgeport.

I drift to sleep recalling familiar forays from earlier years—this true-west country isn't far from home for us, after all. Hydro, Hext, Texola, we'll catch you on another day.

For now, the memory of the Ribbon Road persists, and perhaps the road will, as well. Only a few days after we'd traversed it, the Miami City Council

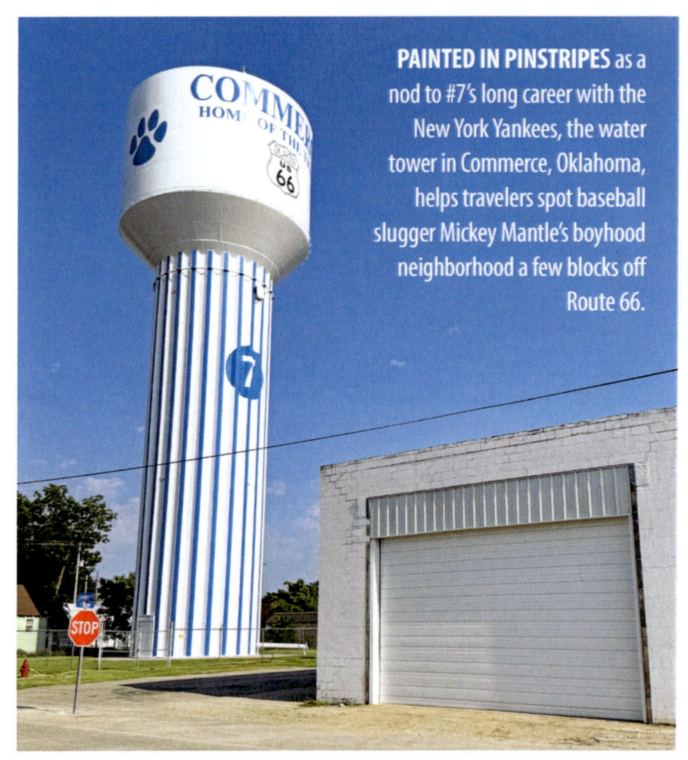

PAINTED IN PINSTRIPES as a nod to #7's long career with the New York Yankees, the water tower in Commerce, Oklahoma, helps travelers spot baseball slugger Mickey Mantle's boyhood neighborhood a few blocks off Route 66.

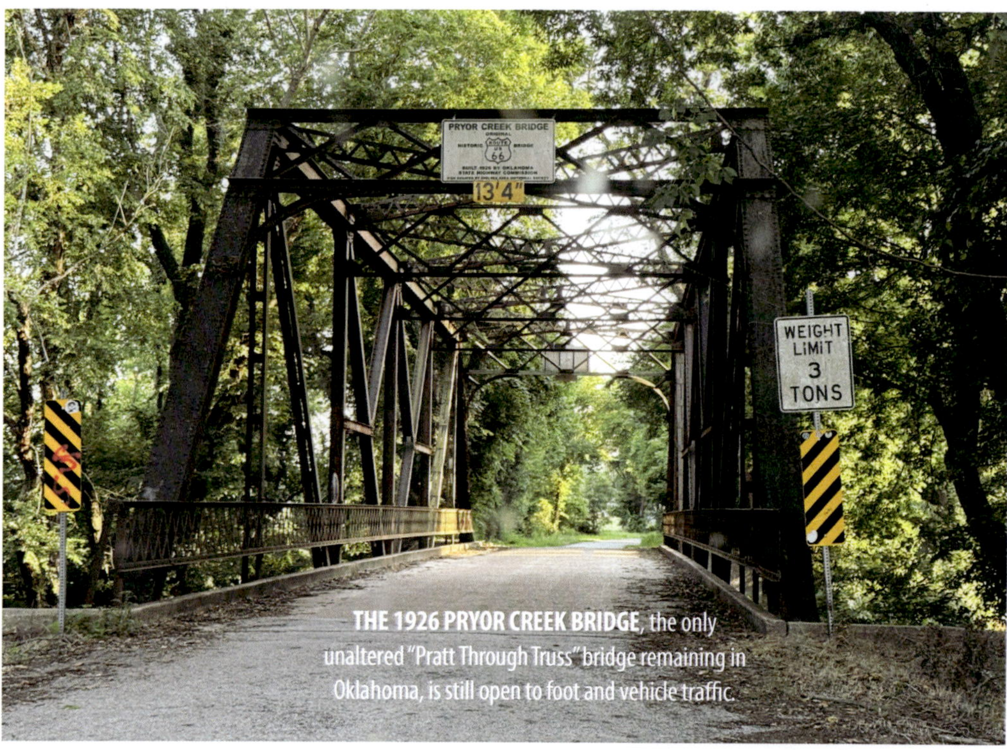

THE 1926 PRYOR CREEK BRIDGE, the only unaltered "Pratt Through Truss" bridge remaining in Oklahoma, is still open to foot and vehicle traffic.

tabled its proposal to grind up and repave the Sidewalk Highway.

"A solution has been reached to keep a century-old historic Ottawa County tourist landmark partially intact," read KSN16's FourStatesHomepage on July 17. The compromise, proposed in a July 16 letter, would leave one mile of the three-mile roadway untouched, said spokesmen for city and county.

"Having that original piece, that attracts tourists from all over. From, you know, all over England and Scotland and Vietnam," Miami mayor Bless Parker told KOAM-TV on July 20. "I mean, I've met people from all over the world, Germany, all over the world that want to come see that piece of the Ribbon Road."

A single mile, hmm.

Perhaps a few more could yet be spared…for those from around the globe, or next door in Texas? Now, where's Woody Guthrie when you need him to compose a tune? ☞

CHAMPION OF THE ROUTE
Tulsa native Rhys Martin, a photographer who became a partisan of Route 66 more than a decade ago, took the reins of the Oklahoma Route 66 Association in 2019. As the 2026 Route centennial approached, he's advocated for funding, signage and wayfinding, and cross-country collaboration. "It's the people (of Route 66) who are really special, who really cement it as an experience."

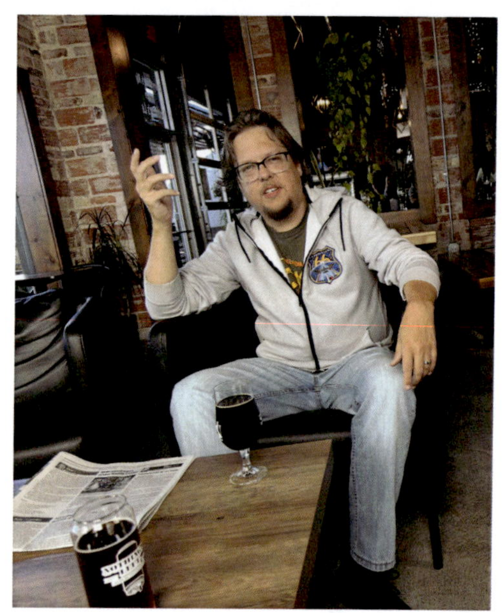

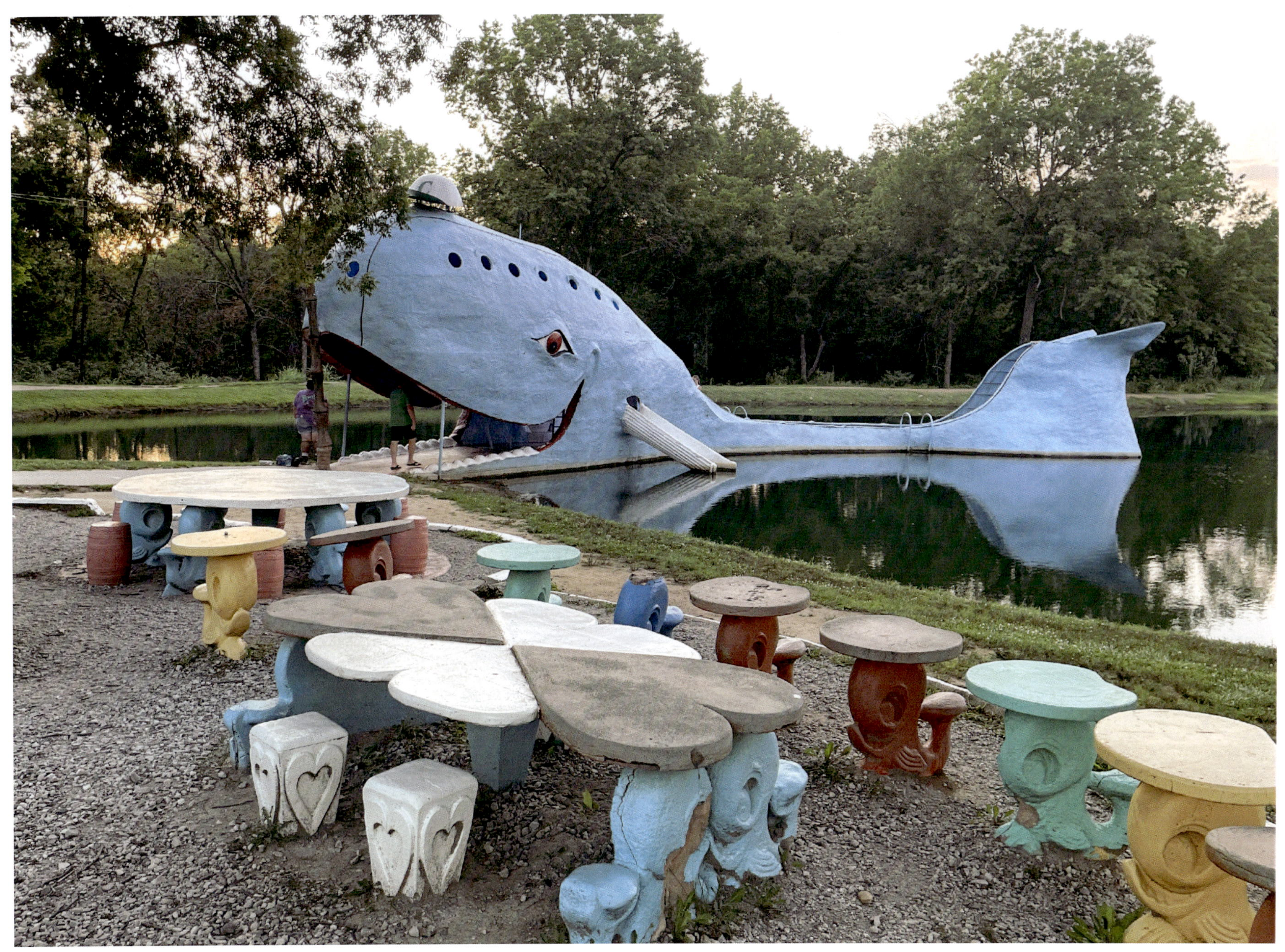

THE BLUE WHALE within view of the Mother Road in Catoosa, Oklahoma, was built in 1972 as a private family swimming spot; it soon opened to the public and, in time, came under the care of the City of Catoosa.

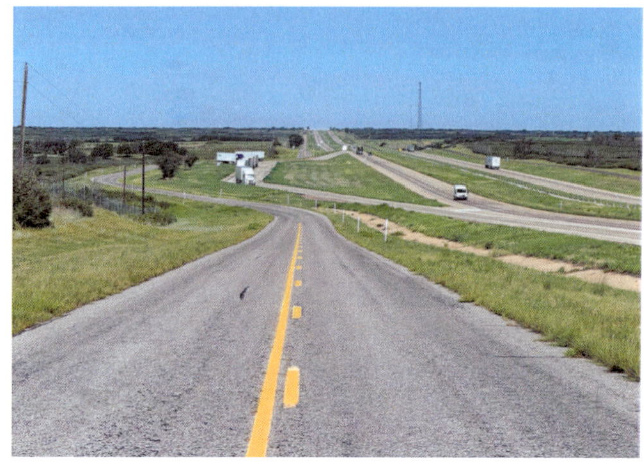

CHAPTER FIVE

Back in Texas—
but not home yet

CROSSING THE STATE LINE WESTBOUND from Oklahoma brings us into familiar territory—not just because it's the state where Kay and I live and make our living, but because it's the start of a very familiar 178 miles of roadway.

From 2012 to 2019 I was privileged to work for the Texas Plains Trail Region, the heritage tourism program of the Texas Historical Commission for the 52 counties of the Plains and Panhandle. It was a mighty cool gig. Promoting economic development and historic preservation in places as far-flung as Amarillo, Benjamin, Canadian, Floydada, Guthrie, Lubbock, Plainview, Post, Slaton—and, yes, Spur—was a huge honor and great fun.

There came a season when preservation of Route 66 as a national historic treasure rose, at last, to the forefront of our program's activism. Legislation to fund the Route 66 Corridor Preservation Program had hit a snag, and preservationists from Illinois to California joined forces to document justifications for keeping the money flowing.

The looming Route 66 centennial, in 2026, was not that far off. A tourism bonanza awaited those communities that could restore and preserve historic gas stations, diners, bridges, patches of roadway, and bits of roadside kitsch, and persuade their highway departments to allow brown-and-white "historic route" waymarking signage bearing the "66" shield.

There came a season when preservation of Route 66 as a national historic treasure rose, at last, to the forefront of our program's activism.

And in Texas, every mile of the state's Route 66 legacy lay in our region. From the Devil's Rope/Route 66 Museum in McLean (housed in a former brassiere-making factory) to the Cadillac Ranch west of Amarillo to the midpoint of the Route in tiny Adrian, supporters banded together. An inventory of assets was made. They included the desolate Jericho Gap stretch of old road from Alanreed to Groom through Donley County, never paved; the well-preserved treasure of commercial buildings in Amarillo's Georgia-to-Western historic district; and the motor courts of Vega, long left to disuse and desolation on the windy high plains.

They also included a unique icon of Route 66 architecture that's inspired imaginations for decades: the U-Drop Inn / Tower Conoco Station in Shamrock.

Today, the U-Drop brings countless drivers and dollars through this community of fewer than 2,000 souls in Wheeler County. It's not a prosperous county; oil and gas, and agriculture, are the primary employers, after the local hospital.

It wasn't a particularly prosperous place in 1936, either, when travelers from points east and west on Route 66 arrived in Shamrock with empty gas tanks and empty stomachs. But a gas-station owner, Tindall, recognized the prospect of increasing automobile traffic at the crossroads of two U.S. highways. A friend used a nail in the dirt to sketch out an art-deco design. When built—including a café and plans for a retail store—it was called

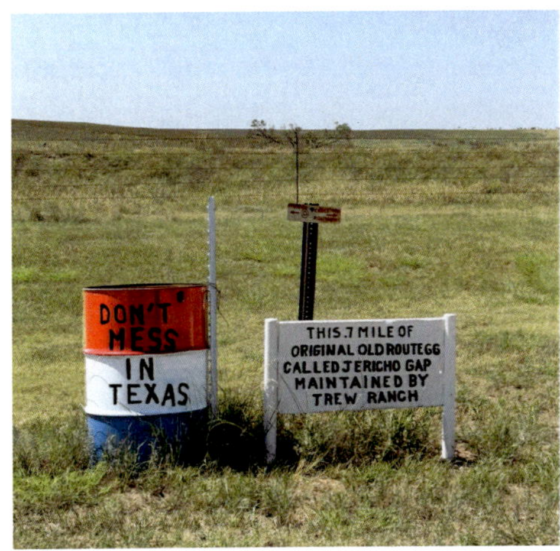

INTREPID TRAVELERS seeking out original, unpaved alignments of Route 66 over the Jericho Gap in Donley County (above) will require detailed maps to avoid private property—and treacherous mud, which wasn't a problem in July 2024.

THE U-DROP INN / CONOCO TOWER (right) welcomes visitors once again from all over the world, after restoration in 2003. After dark its green and pink neon lights are a photographer's delight; here, at midday in July, the bleached-out sky required Photoshopping.

THE SLUG BUG RANCH newly installed at the Big Texan RV Park east of Amarillo (below) bookends the Cadillac Ranch west of the city.

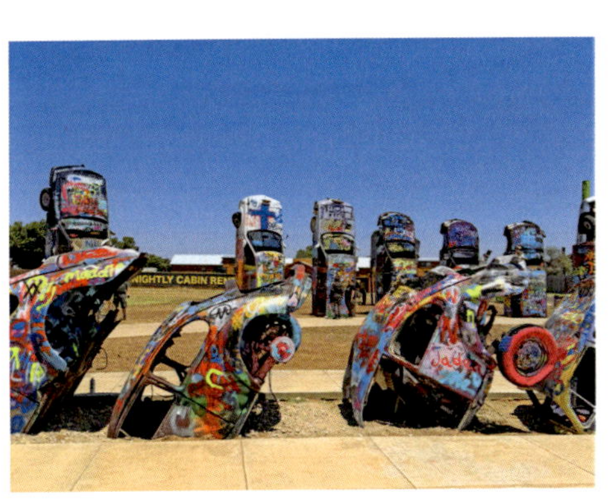

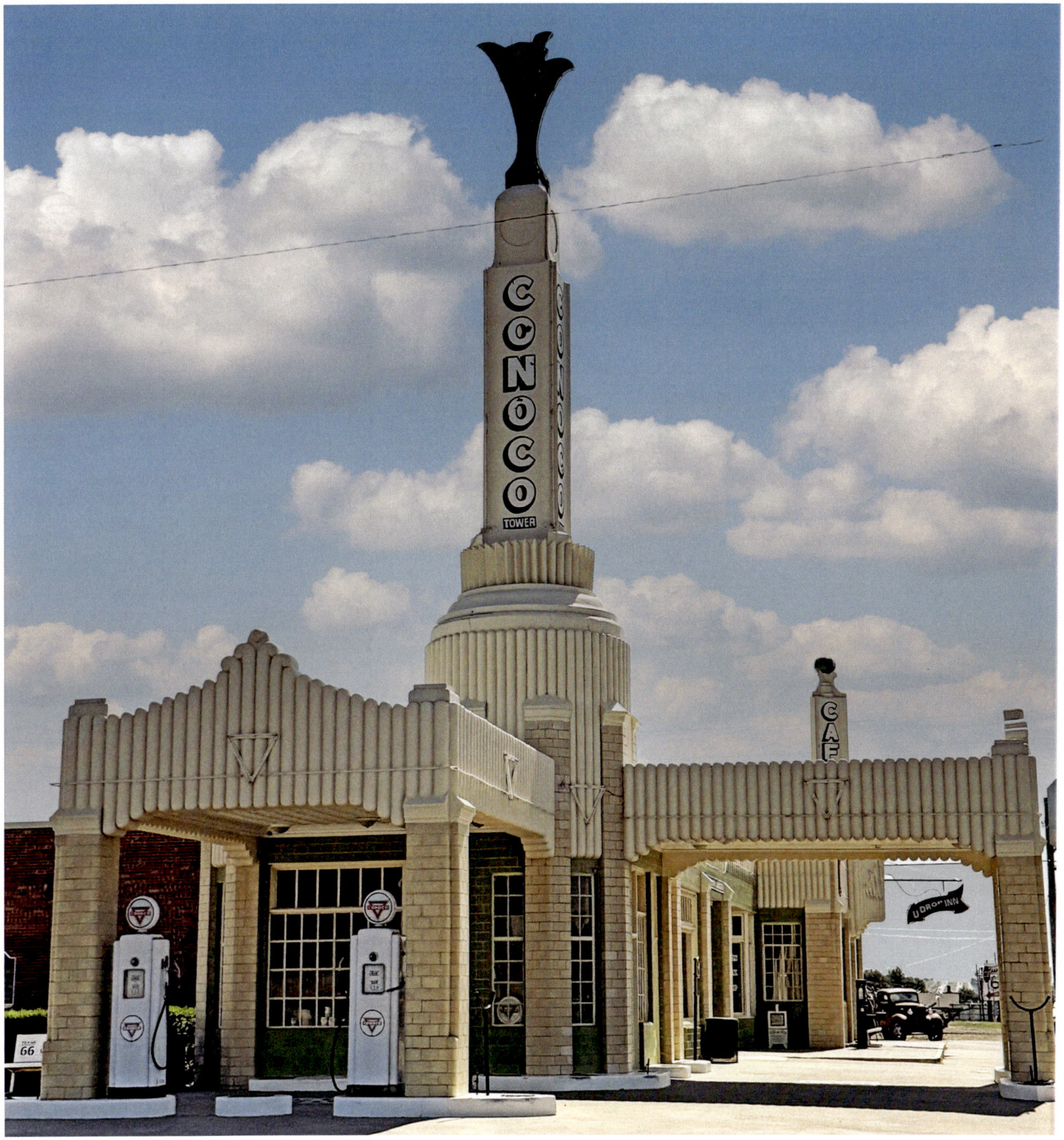

by newspapers "the most up-to-date edifice of its kind on U.S. Highway 66 between Oklahoma City and Amarillo."

Like so many Route 66 inspirations, in due time the structure, with its lime-green neon tubing and distinctive tulip-shaped tower, fell into decline and receivership, prompted primarily by the diversion of traffic to the nearly parallel Interstate 40.

I had first dropped in at the U-Drop twenty-one years ago, in early July 2003.

The *New York Times* regional newspaper for which I was writing my way across the country was the Wilmington (N.C.) *Star-News,* eastern terminus of I-40.

I'd happened into the station as finishing touches were being put in place ahead of its grand reopening.

"Route 66 was still a dirt road here when the U-Drop Inn was built," said then Chamber of Commerce president David Rushing. The inn would soon reopen as an official Texas rest area and an information office for Shamrock.

The route through Shamrock wasn't exactly bustling on that scorching July afternoon, though. Dolores Hibdon, secretary for an auto-towing outfit down the street, described to me the old highway back when her family traveled frequently between California and Oklahoma. "I remember spending the night in Shamrock," she said, pointing westward up the road toward one of the vacant mom-and-pop motels.

"All of that ended when I-40 came through," she pronounced with a sweeping gesture. "They murdered the Mother Road."

Happily for Shamrock, the U-Drop Inn and other restoration projects—plus an enormous boost from the *Cars* movie, which echoed its design in the fictional Ramone's House of Body Art—have brought fame and fortune back to the town, to some degree.

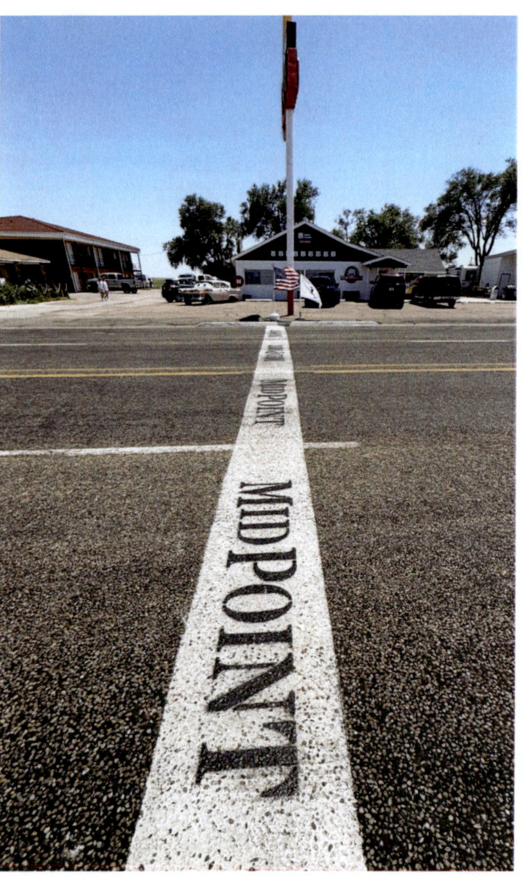

MIDPOINT At Adrian, Texas—23 miles from the New Mexico state line—Route 66 through-travelers from either direction are midway through their journey.

Past the icons of Texas' Panhandle ranching country, including the straight-and-narrow giant cross and the leaning water tower at Groom, the rising framework of the next Buc-cee's across from Amarillo's Texas Travel Information Center, and the enticements of the Big Texan Steak Ranch's 72-Ounce Steak Challenge, we're eager to abandon necessary portions of I-40 once more for the Mother Road.

Its own mother, at least within the aforementioned mile-long U.S. Route 66-Sixth Street Historic District in Amarillo, is a petite bundle of energy who drives a sunshine-hued MG roadster dubbed "The Yellow Imposter."

Dora Meroney began championing Route 66 in the late 1990s, when she and her mother opened an antiques store in the family home, a brick bungalow situated directly on the Route.

"You have to make your street look nice, and make sure it has something visitors want to see when they get here," Meroney had told me for a magazine piece in 2018.

Meroney practices what she preaches: whenever visitors stop by, as they do daily from around the globe, they're invited to have their likeness posted to the shop's Facebook, with Texas Ivy's Route 66 shield as a backdrop.

Meroney wasn't in her shop the day we made our own return to her block of Route 66. But the historic district was bustling—jam-packed on a Saturday with diners, bookshop patrons, sidewalk strollers, antiques hunters, bikers, buskers, curiosity-seekers.

At the western end of the mile stands the completed project Meroney and her buddies brought to fruition just last year. The enormous blue water tower at 6th and Western boasts a brand-new coat of paint—and an Amarillo Route 66 shield. The landmark beckons, drawing traffic off the thoroughfares and onto this stretch of the Route unparalleled for its shoulder-to-shoulder historic structures and its cadre of shopkeeps and supporters.

It's too dang hot to even think about trudging, spray paint can in hand, out to the pasture-planted array of rusted autos known as the Cadillac Ranch, just west of Amarillo. We've done it dozens of times before, anyway. Yet here it is a hundred degrees at noon, and the I-40 access road is lined for a hundred yards in either direction with visitors' vehicles.

So instead we speed ahead via the Interstate to a place where dessert awaits the faithful. If it feels like cheating, well, we're no strangers to every driveable mile that parallels this stretch (I have documented actual mileposts, in all seasons). We rejoin the old pavement at Vega, where I'm pleased to see how the Milburn-Price Culture Museum has come along since its start in 2015, and that Rooster's is still serving up calf fries (hey, someone's got to).

But the delicacy for which people travel half the distance of the Route is the pie at the Midpoint Café. Tiny Adrian doubles its population daily with diners desirous of this delicacy, and its other deli delights.

Kay and I select from among the rustic-crust desserts. Even at midafternoon, the converted gas station is packed, with owner Brenda Hammit hustling about like a mother hen tending to a flock. Though she didn't invent the Ugly Crust Pie (credit former owner Fran Houser with that innovation), she carries on the tradition with gusto.

Among the satisfied patrons today are *Route* Magazine publisher Brennen Matthews and his family, on their own sightseeing tour. They drive from their Toronto hometown across the U.S. each summer, he said, and they've found a niche in publishing the slick color book that we've spotted on the welcome-counter stand here and all across our journey.

We see he's got his own interviews to conduct, and we bid them a fond farewell. Everyone is out making new memories and following the myriad old stories along this well-worn route.

"Maybe we'll catch up with you along the way!"

Outside in the searing heat, it's almost—*almost*—possible to imagine the cool things and cooler weather that might await just over the rise. New Mexico's Blue Hole, Tucumcari neon, mountains and mesas. The dusky colors of Arizona's Painted Desert. We can almost smell California from here.

Sugar-sated, we snap a quick pic at the midpoint line across the highway, jump back into the black pickup.

Halfway. Half the story told, half to go. ☞

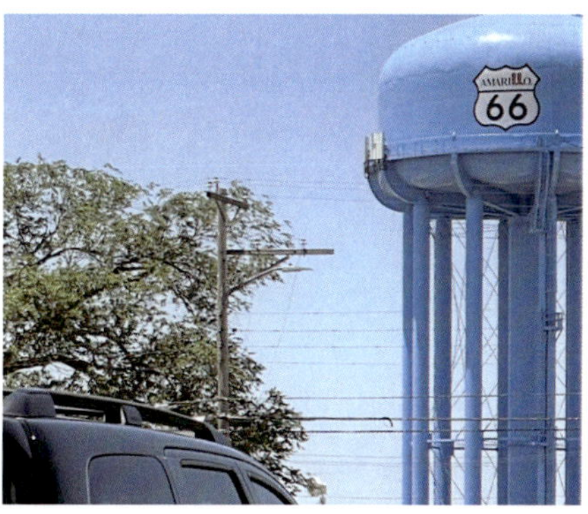

AMARILLO'S WATER TOWER guides drivers to the historic retail district between Georgia and Western. The project was a local triumph in 2023.

BRENDA AND BRENNEN talk turkey about Route 66 travel at her Midpoint Café in Adrian, Texas.

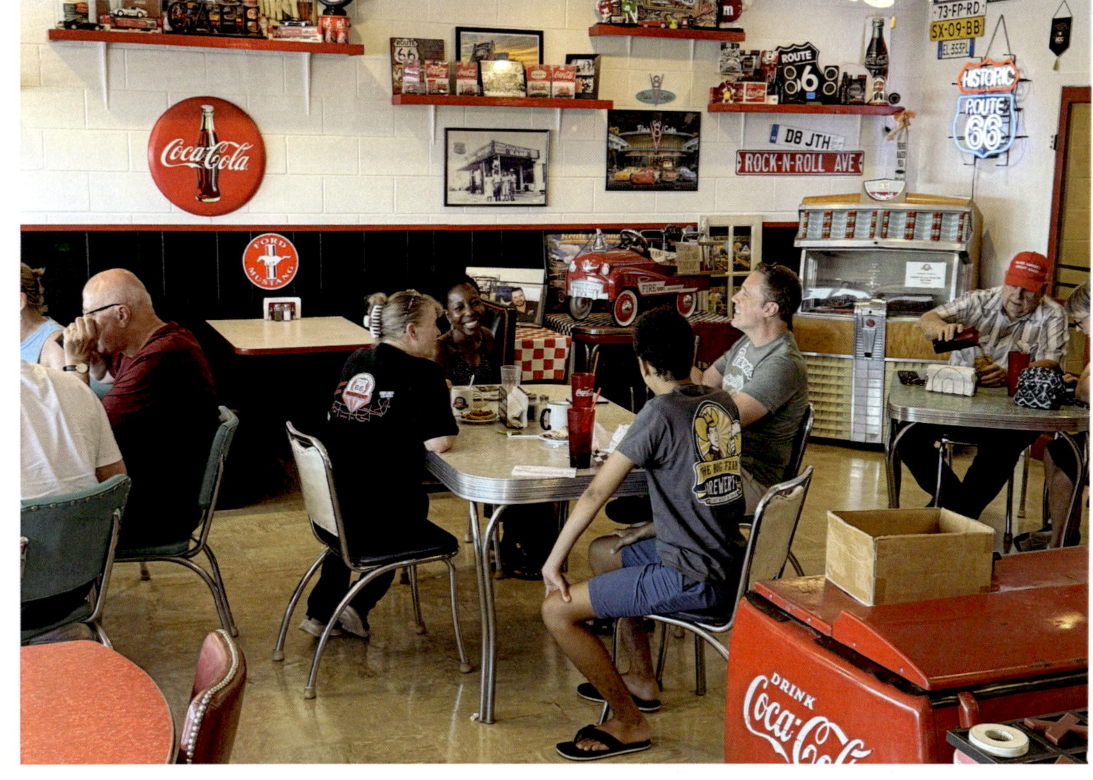

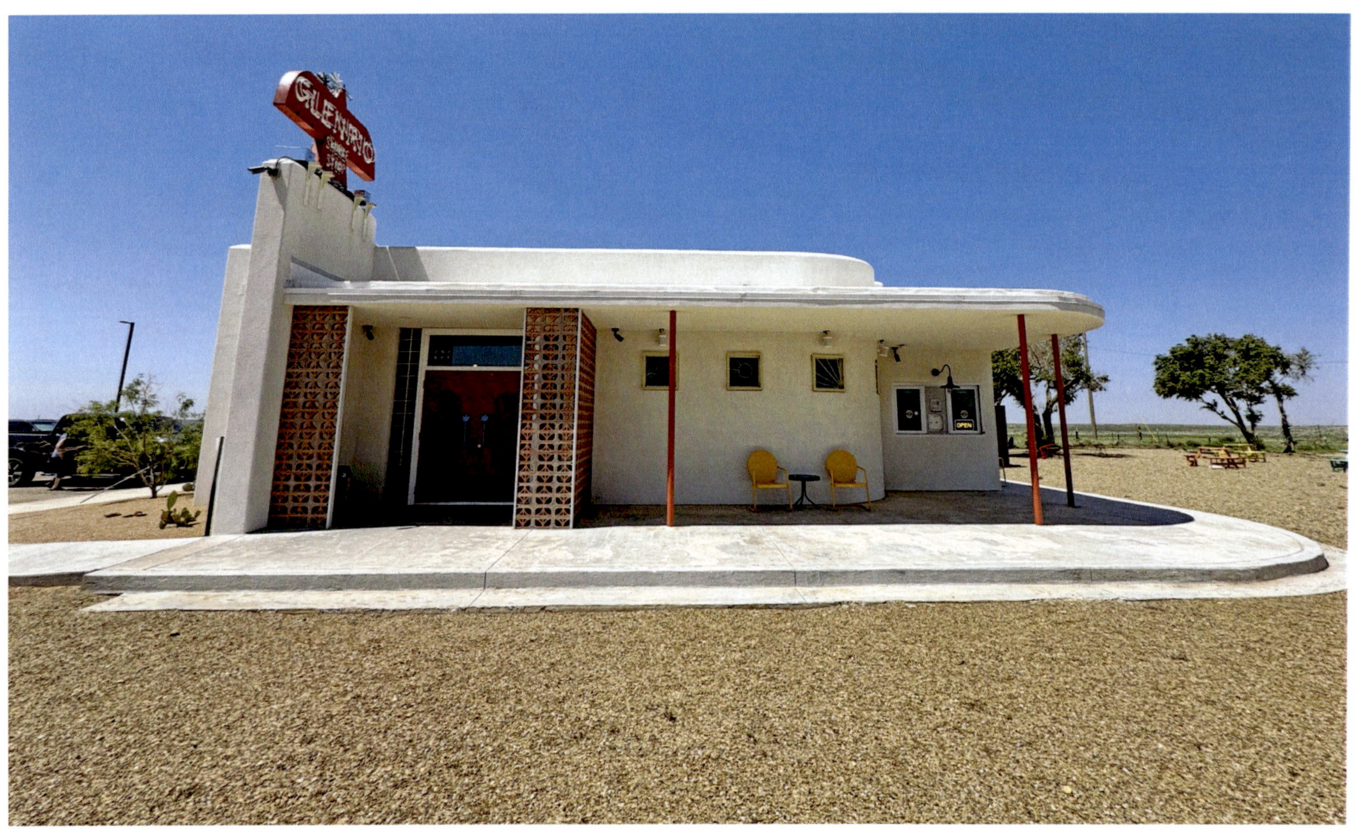

HIGH DESERT At Glenrio, a town that once straddled the New Mexico–Texas line, the Glenrio Smoke Shop has supplanted the site once occupied by the old post office.

EXIT ZERO FOR GLENRIO to find yourself in the "high" desert at the Texas–New Mexico line.

A JULY MIDAFTERNOON is not the time to idle for miles in an I-40 traffic jam. We bypassed that stretch of Route 66 instead.

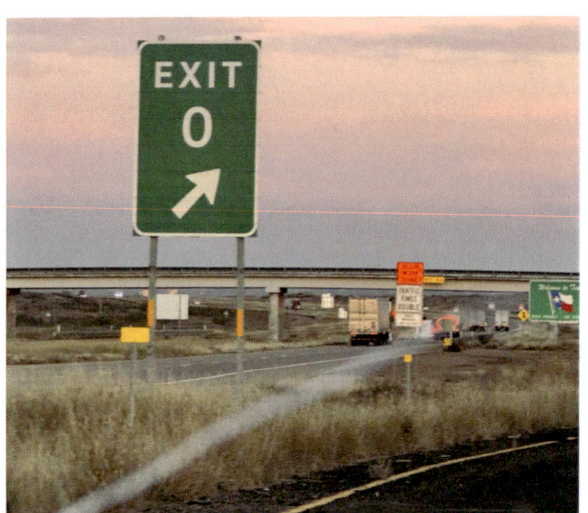

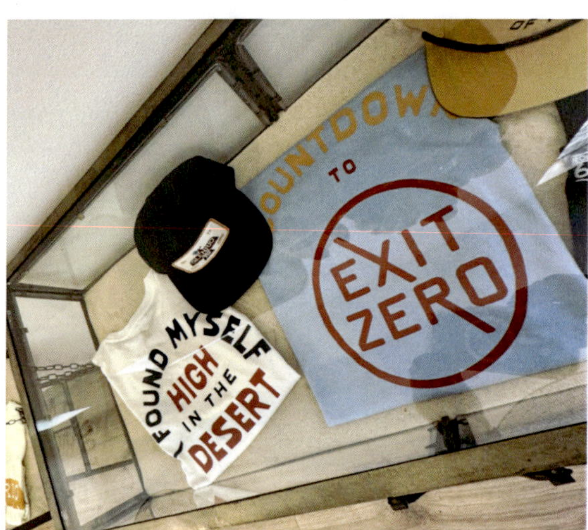

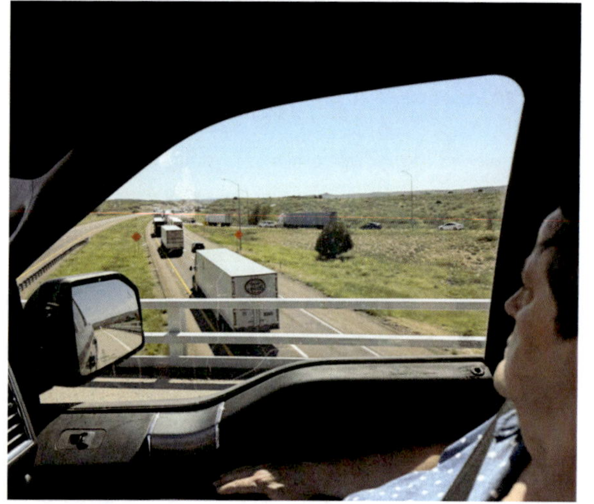

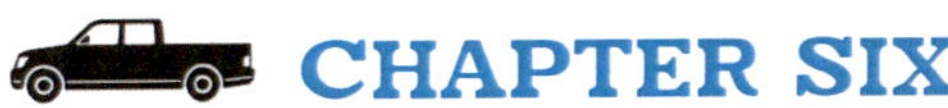

CHAPTER SIX

Route 66 through New Mexico: Light across the high desert

New Mexico likes to call itself the Land of Enchantment.

And so it is, quite often, for their next-door neighbors the Texans in particular. We come here often.

The two states' kinship stretches back a good ways—to the era when both were parts of old Mexico, and before that, the domain of nomadic or settled indigenous tribes.

But there truly is, to my way of thinking, something tantalizing and magnetic about the quality of light and color in the New Mexico landscape. I sense it every time I drive west over the line from mesquite to juniper, at the diffuse western edge of the Llano Estacado plateau.

Along historic Route 66—little of which remains unscathed by I-40 in the eastern part of New Mexico—that change starts to become apparent at the Texas–New Mexico line, in the ghost town of Glenrio.

Glenrio never numbered but about a hundred souls in its long-ago heyday. The stop on the Rock Island

New Mexico likes to call itself the Land of Enchantment. And so it is, quite often, for their next-door neighbors the Texans.

Railroad in the early 20th century soon offered fuel on the Texas side for motorists on the Ozark Trail—an unpaved precursor to Route 66—and mail delivery on the New Mexico side (the mail sacks were brought to it for distribution from Texas). By the twenty-first century, the fast lanes of I-40 had long since siphoned off most of Glenrio's residents. By the year 2000, according to the Handbook of Texas Online, citizens numbered precisely five.

The motel and gas station on the Texas side, and the café and post office on the New Mexico side, had been left to the considerable extremes of the elements. But green returned in 2021—as greenback dollars, and as newly legalized cannabis.

On a prominence overlooking the constant river of Interstate traffic, the Glenrio Smoke Stop rises like a white-stucco chapel. A red eagle sign beckons; a handsomely landscaped parking area and patio contrast dramatically with the ruin rampant elsewhere in the erstwhile town.

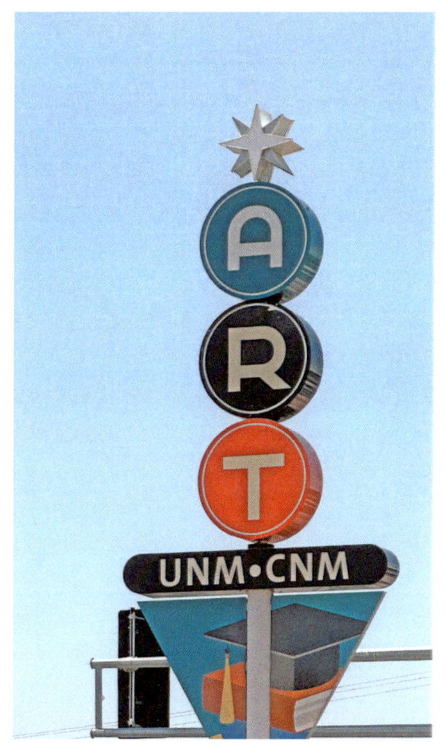

ART IN ABQ The landscape and highway-scape of northern New Mexico, through which historic Route 66 passes, lends itself at every turn to the work of painters, sculptors, architects, writers, dancers—and even bus drivers. (This sign marking an Albuquerque Rapid Transit stop on Central Avenue—old 66—fits right in.)

Turns out the dispensary business thrives here, far from any other population except that of I-40—which, according to TxDOT's 2024 count, amounted to some 15,000 vehicles daily. Friendly staff inside the shop's clean, well-lighted, spa-like space assist customers from near and far with an array of weed products, and with up-to-date information on what can be transported where. It's a far sight from how this hamlet must have looked a hundred years ago. But maybe things haven't really changed that much; back in the 1930s, it was alcohol that could be purchased at Glenrio's New Mexico saloon, while over the line Texas was dry.

A short distance west lies Tucumcari, where the attractions shift from green to blue. In 2024, knowing that the famous Blue Swallow Motel and its gloriously-hued neon palette had changed hands a few times in recent years, we'd stopped in, reservationless, for a quick look.

Hosts Robert and Dawn Federico invited us back for a longer stay, and we promised to make good on the offer—especially to stay at a place where the owner insists on providing a cup of coffee for two travelers who aren't even paying guests yet.

A year later the opportunity arose. The impromptu chance to attend a media conference in Salt Lake City occurred during the fall 2025 shutdown of the U.S. government. While the unfortunate circumstance would prevent hoped-for visits to national parks and historic sites (more about that later), it also, more happily, forced us to choose driving over air travel.

And we knew exactly where we wanted to spend our first night on the road. We crossed

fingers—and were delighted, on short notice, to book the Lillian Redman suite at the Blue Swallow.

Then, departure morning of our ten-day trip began with a setback: Kay took a scary fall off the back porch before sunup, injuring her shin and ankle and suffering a half-inch gash at her hairline. After cold compress, bandages, and Advil, she determined to forge ahead.

Never were we so glad to encounter such touches of vintage luxury as those afforded by the Blue Swallow. Pulling in at dusk with picnic sandwiches and more ice compresses in the cooler, we had only to back the Acadia into the adjoining garage, then settle into the lawn chairs under the stars and soak up the evening breeze. No pinging elevators, no long corridors, no plastic keys to swipe. Awestruck voices of arriving motorists; the pastel palette of light and sky; and the prospect of awaiting clawfoot tub, luxurious bathrobes, soft carpets and chenille bed coverings was like a mix of vacation spa and Grandma's house. A good night's sleep in the suite named for the Blue Swallow's resident spirit was restorative for body and soul.

We hang around till midmorning for a cruise of Tucumcari's many mid-century landmarks. Indications of restoration in advance of the Route centennial were everywhere, not only along the main drag but downtown—an often overlooked treasure. Only the city's western fringe showed no sign of new life.

We take our time, consulting maps for old pavement, but recent rains have flooded out numerous low-water crossings and we're forced back to I-40. On the home stretch we plan to follow that pre-1937 alignment via Santa Fe, and perhaps

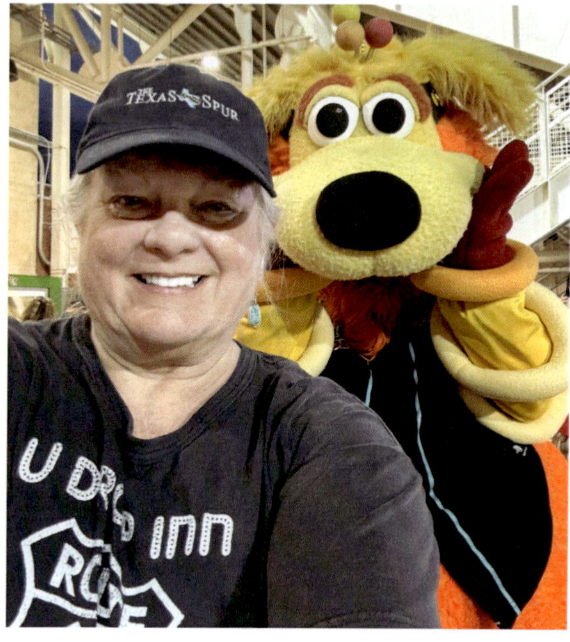

ORBIT (at right, not the figure in the Texas Spur cap) is the wacky mascot of the Albuquerque Isotopes baseball team, the only franchise in professional sports to get its name from a "Simpsons" TV episode.

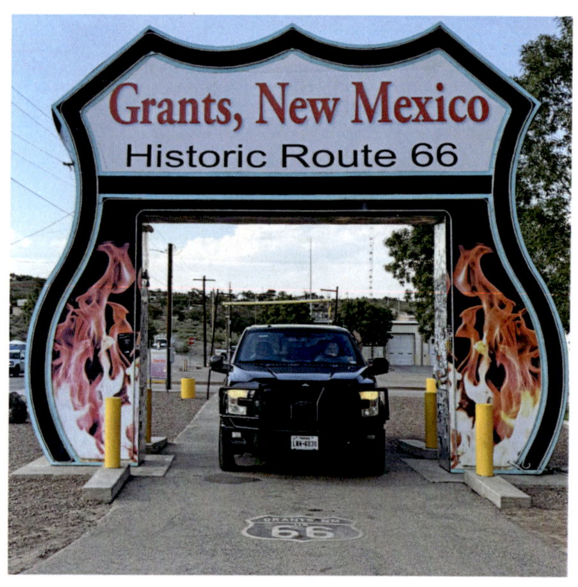

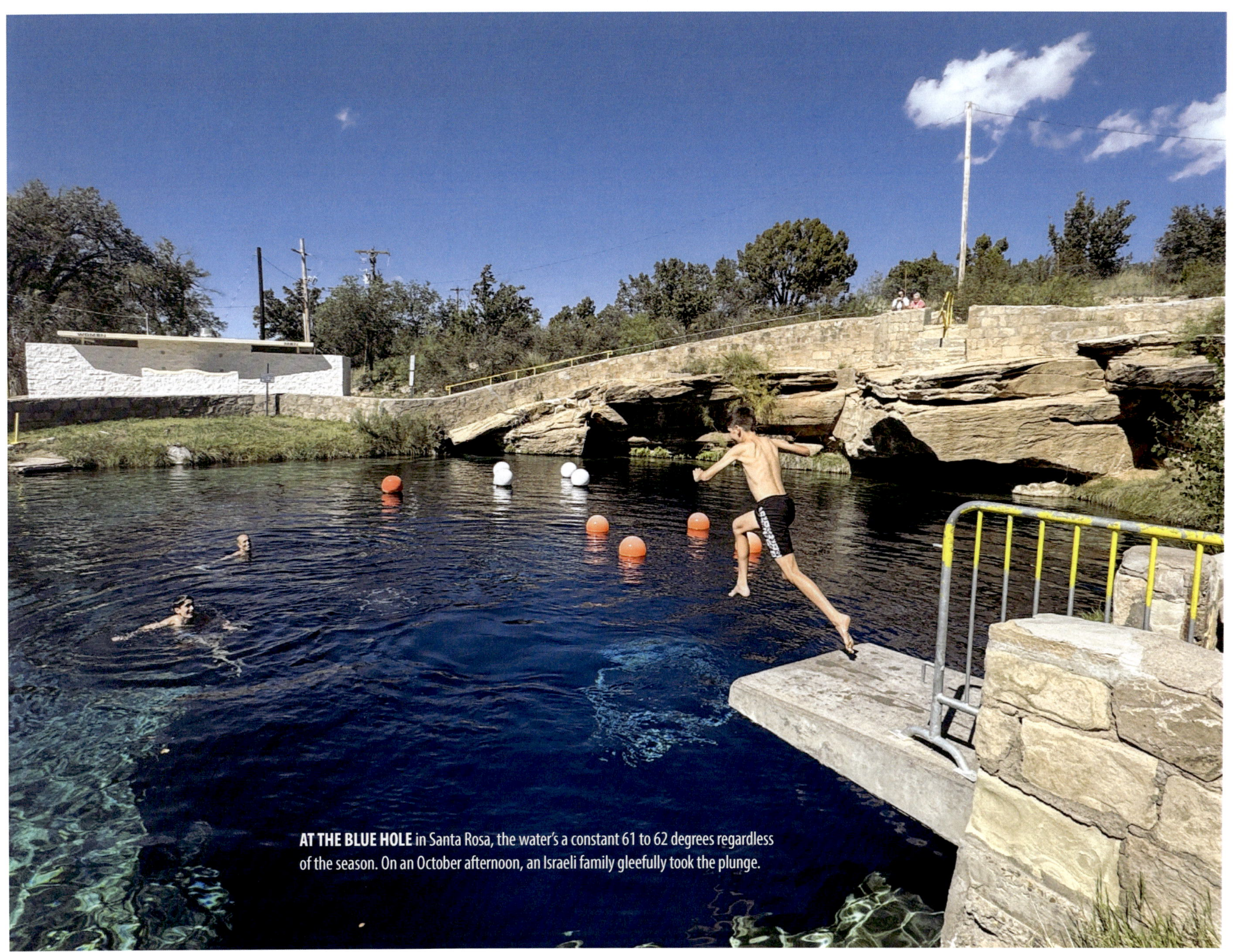

AT THE BLUE HOLE in Santa Rosa, the water's a constant 61 to 62 degrees regardless
of the season. On an October afternoon, an Israeli family gleefully took the plunge.

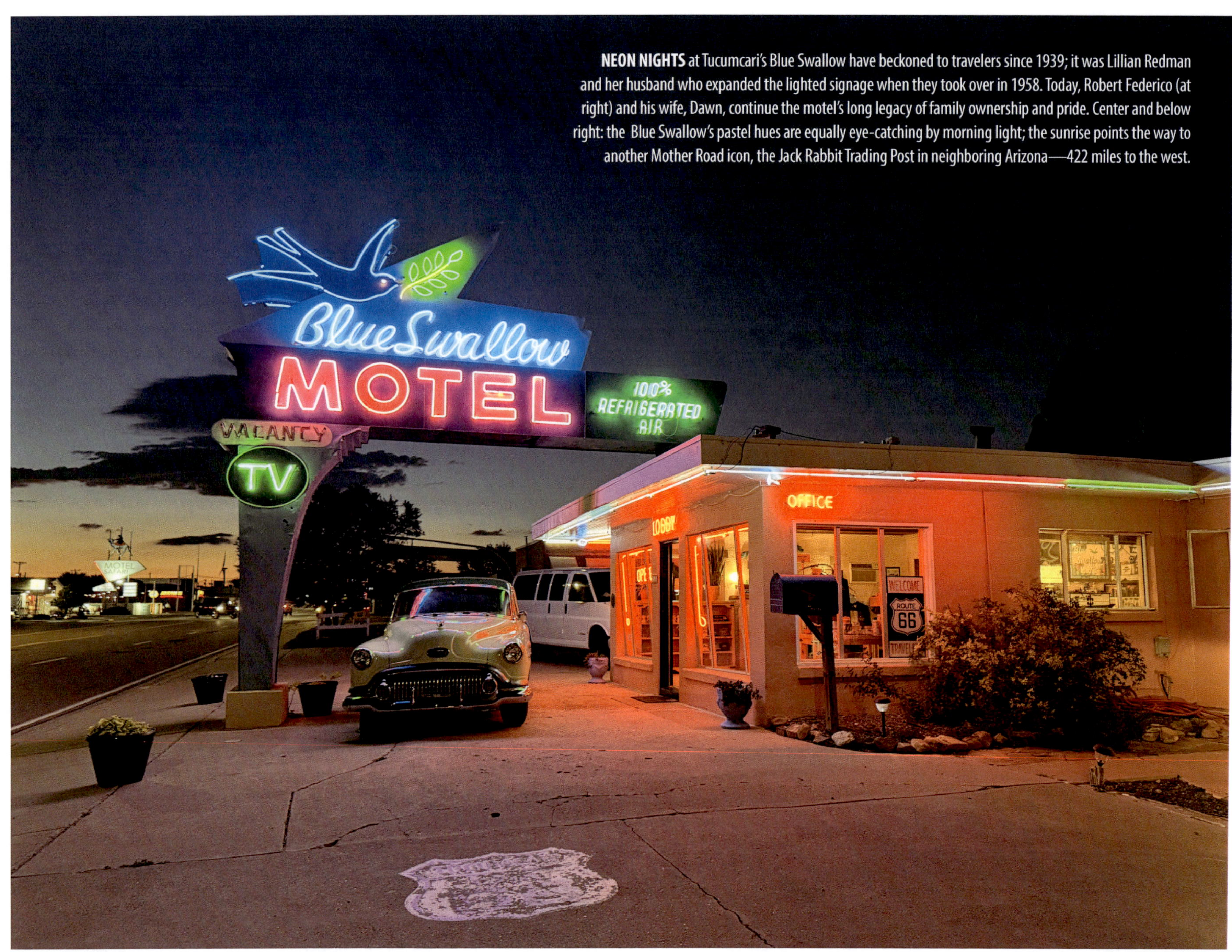

NEON NIGHTS at Tucumcari's Blue Swallow have beckoned to travelers since 1939; it was Lillian Redman and her husband who expanded the lighted signage when they took over in 1958. Today, Robert Federico (at right) and his wife, Dawn, continue the motel's long legacy of family ownership and pride. Center and below right: the Blue Swallow's pastel hues are equally eye-catching by morning light; the sunrise points the way to another Mother Road icon, the Jack Rabbit Trading Post in neighboring Arizona—422 miles to the west.

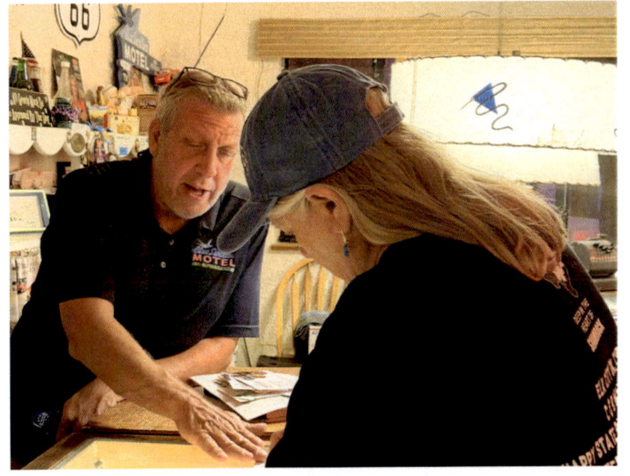

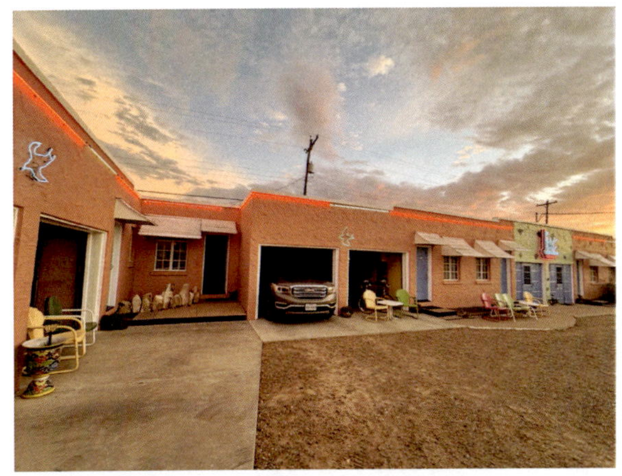

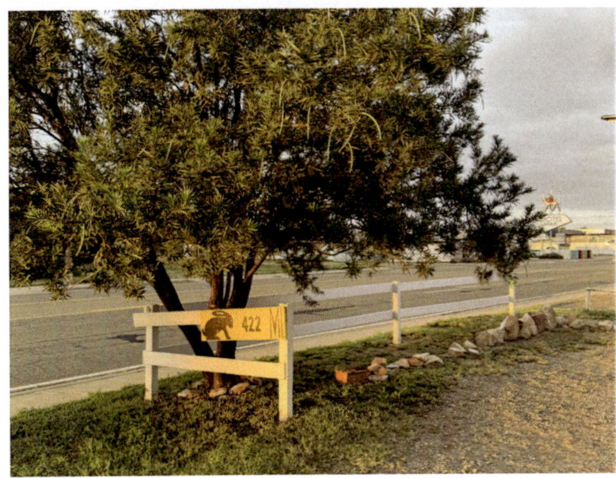

some of these roads will be passable again a week hence.

To our north and south, beyond the dry, mounded hills adorned with low juniper and piñon lie vast ranches, irrigated fields, lonely two-lanes. Ahead lie the mountains. Over the Sandia range that spills us out of I-40's high-speed roller-coaster, we're finally able to rejoin Route 66 in its colorful role as the main drag of Albuquerque, Central Avenue.

With its arrow-straight trajectory down into the "bowl" of the Rio Grande, Central limns a captivating picture of Route 66 even if a traveler never ventures off it. From the once-inviting hotels of the International District on the east side (many of which have been converted to shelter for the unhoused population) to the trendy eateries of Nob Hill and the diners and dives of the University of New Mexico neighborhood, to Old Town and the splendidly restored El Vado motor court near Tingley Beach, it's impossible to absorb enough of Albuquerque's varied vistas in a single visit. Plan on a week here if you want to sample blue-corn tortillas, visit a terrific bookstore, stroll the bosque, ride the aerial tramway, or suss out the car wash from *Breaking Bad.*

On last summers visit we'd detoured a few blocks south to take in a game at the city's ballpark, home of the minor-league Albuquerque Isotopes. We'd snagged tickets to one of the special-promotion nights when the team plays as Los Mariachis de Nuevo México, and the lowriders on display, the spiffy turquoise jerseys and bright plastic bobbleheads, and frozen margaritas combine with "Llévame al juego de beisbol" sung during the seventh-inning stretch for a fun evening in the grandstands.

My own son completed his studies in art here at UNM, so perhaps I am already inclined to think of the state in visual-art terms. Moody as a Peter Hurd composition, flat and delineated as a Baumann woodcut, bright and blended as an O'Keeffe, backlit as a Blumenschein, angular and layered as an Abeyta canvas: the hues and textures of this state surround us everywhere we go.

While the galleries and museums of Santa Fe are where many art lovers gravitate, I've always found the university's art museum in Albuquerque inspiring and usually uncrowded—and it's free. It houses the largest collection of art in New Mexico. Plus, it's only steps away from the Route and close enough for a lunch stop at the funky Frontier Restaurant for a carne adovada burrito.

After a couple hours' layover in the Duke City to check on our week's newspaper issues, we're ready to hit the road again for parts unknown. Historic Route 66 weaves through parts of Western New Mexico's Colorado Plateau that are home to Puebloan cultures—Acoma, Laguna—and the Navajo Nation.

We traverse the blacktop westward wherever we can keep track of it.

That indescribable light is a tractor beam pulling us onward. In the small city of Grants, sunset hues reflected off pastels, neon and space-age angles. But an unexpected delight awaited us in an otherwise unremarkable city park. Fiberglass reflector dishes from the satellite TV era lined the highway—repainted with traditional, geometric

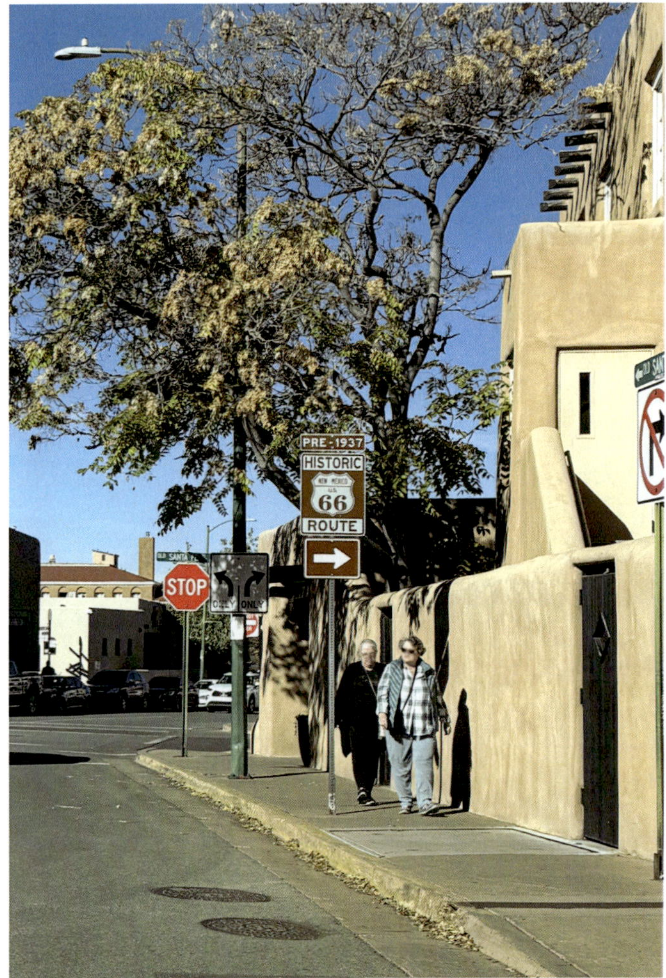

PRE-1937 ROUTE took travelers into northern New Mexico's mountain passes through Santa Fe, the oldest state capital in the United States. On a return trip in October 2025, we traced the route eastbound across the old Santa Fe Trail to Las Vegas, New Mexico and southeast to connect with I-40 again at Tucumcari.

BASKET CASE In Grants, an array of repurposed satellite dishes installed in 2018 projects the beauty of native designs, including this Jicarilla Apache example in a half-mile-long "windshield museum" worth stopping to learn more about.

native basket designs. A more perfect repurposing of eyesore into art I may never have witnessed.

While much of New Mexico, from its trendy galleries to the Indian markets of Gallup, is known for its exhibits and sales, it doesn't take a bankroll to appreciate art throughout the length of the state's Route 66 miles. It's right there on public display for free, as public murals, mosaics, sculptures, architecture.

As our multi-day trek across the Land of Enchantment began with the subtle pastels of the east, it deepened into brilliant hues of Albuquerque's Central Avenue nightscape, and has now burnished to gold and turquoise in the sunset over Gallup.

The highlighted neon sign at the famous El Rancho Hotel, where the stars once came out to the desert for movie shoots, buzzes on. While the hotel's paying guests pull up and park, then roll their suitcases in to gawk at the lobby's Hollywood memorabilia, we pause a second to snap our photos and then pop the Ford into gear again. We cruise the hillsides of the city, windows down, searching out cameos of golden-hour glimmer. A muffler man from a Route 66 heyday stands guard on a rooftop. Down in the valley, where the rail lines run, the famous old Harvey House inn remains as a reminder of glamour days. Pinks and purples vie for prominence in the east as oranges sink below the western horizon.

Sometimes the best gallery show is right there, for free. ☞

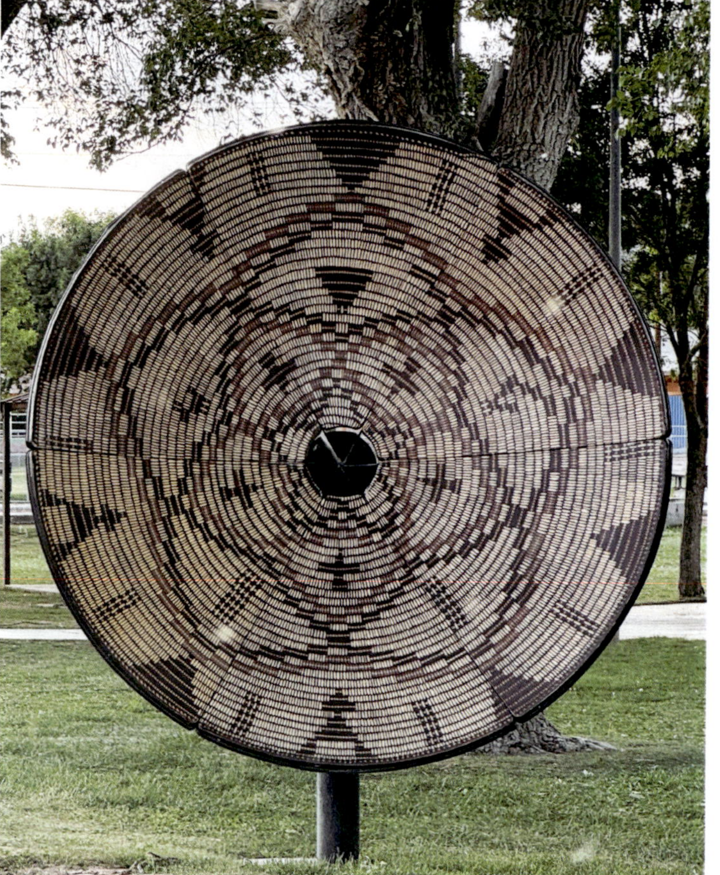

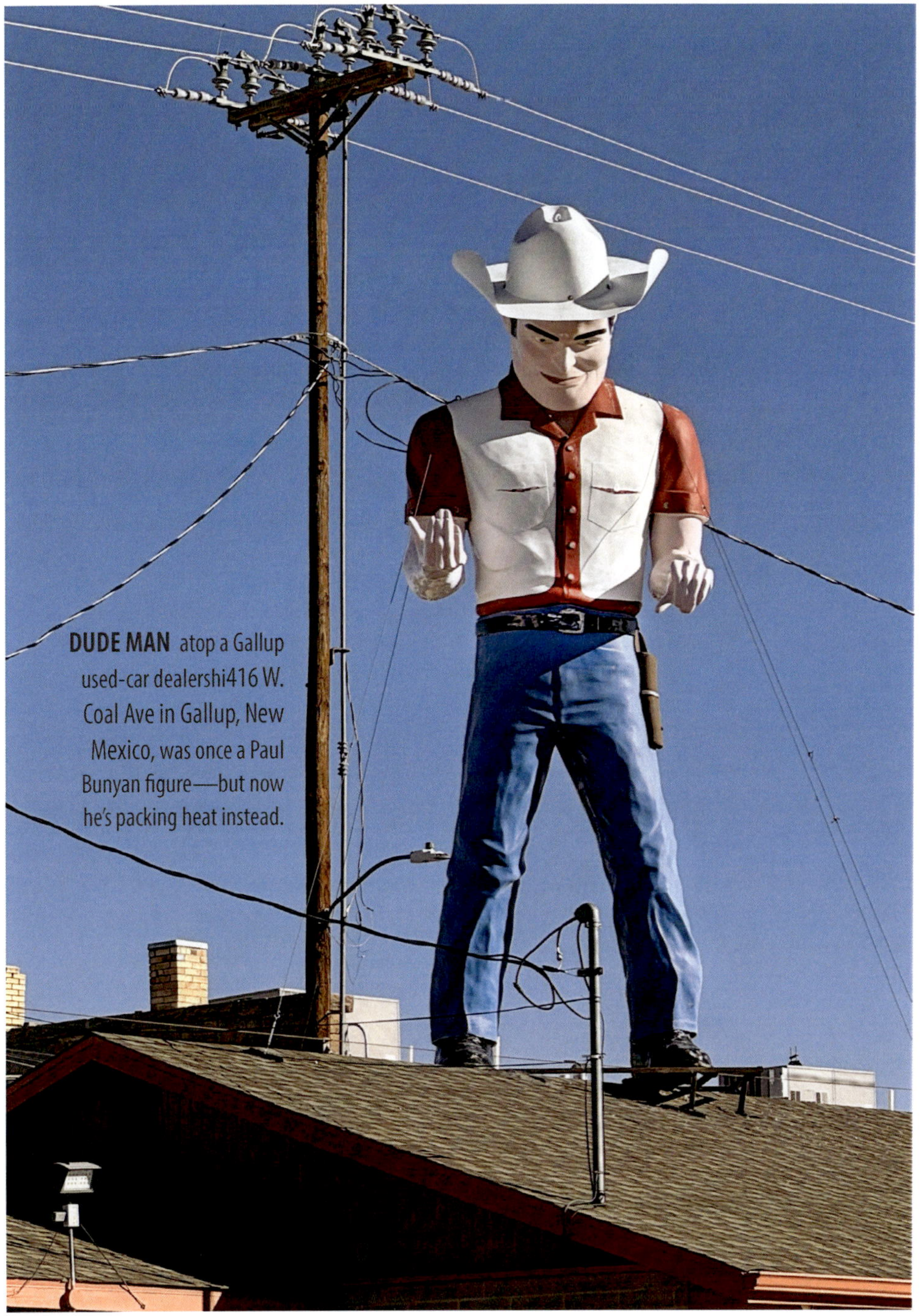

DUDE MAN atop a Gallup used-car dealershi416 W. Coal Ave in Gallup, New Mexico, was once a Paul Bunyan figure—but now he's packing heat instead.

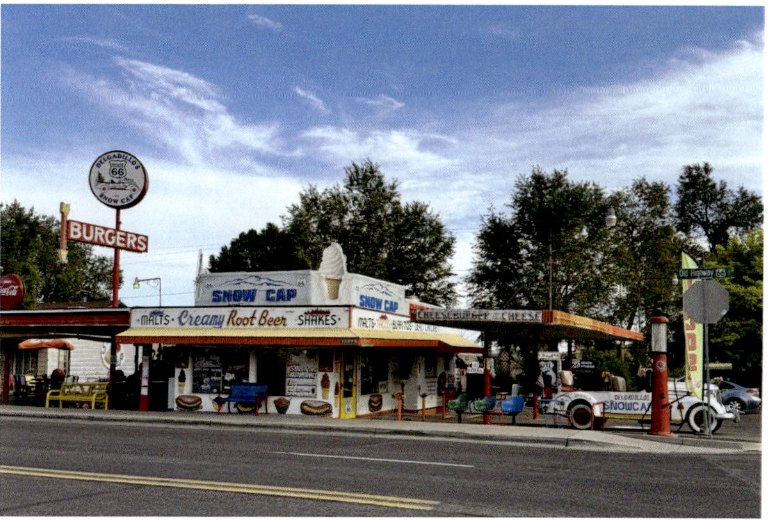

SORRY, WE'RE *NOT* OPEN Both times we passed through Seligman, Arizona, we missed Route roadie Angel Delgadillo, whose barbershop was closed for the day—but we snapped a colorful shot of the invitingly cool Snow Cap Drive-in, founded by Angel's late brother Juan in 1953.

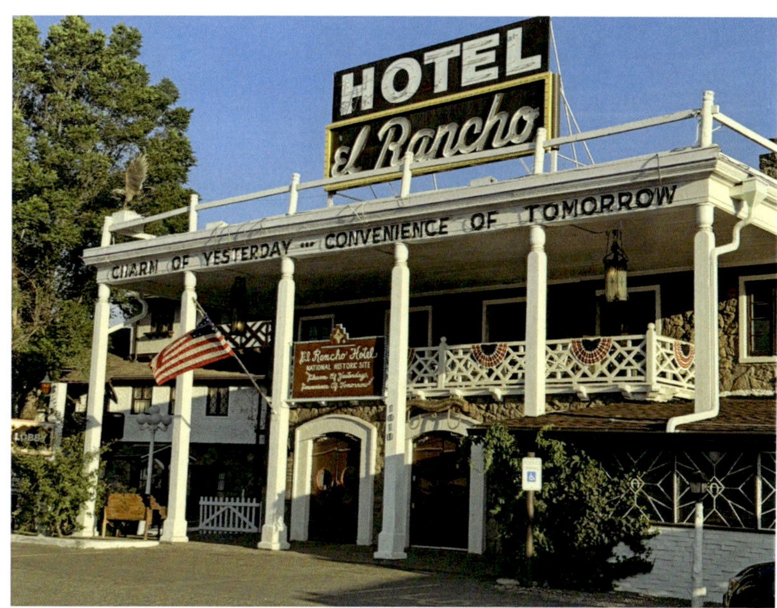

HOTEL EL RANCHO preserves the "Charm of Yesterday" while providing the "Convenience of Tomorrow" in downtown Gallup—since 1936.

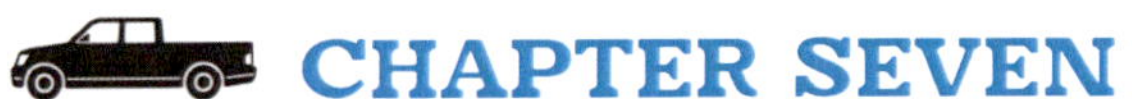

CHAPTER SEVEN

Animals all across Arizona

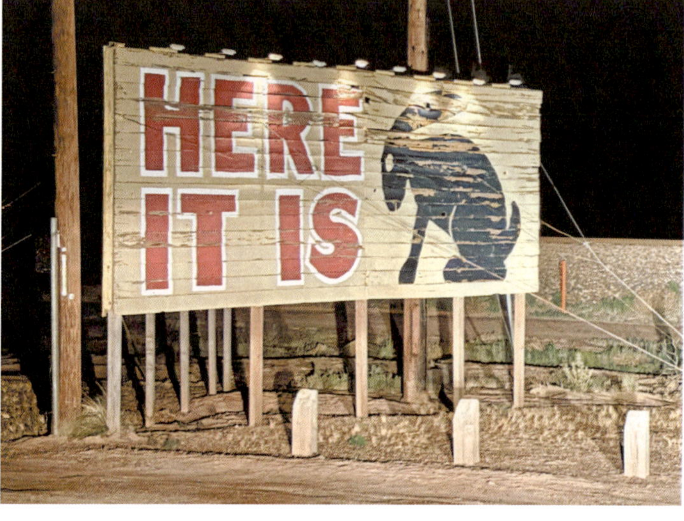

Arriving at the eastern edge of Arizona at dusk during our summer 2024 traverse means two things: that the 149 miles between here and Flagstaff will zoom past in darkness; and that we'll see precious little of Mother Road pavement on this stretch.

As the guidebooks tell us, "the old road is effectively submerged beneath the freeway" in the eastern two-thirds of the state. Our first pulloff, however, brings us to the unmistakable tourist draw of Chief Yellowhorse's cave.

Here, twenty-one years ago as an Easterner, I spied my first-ever live bison. The buffalo were penned in a large enclosure in the shadow of the enormous rock ledge. I took a photo with my Kodak—an early digital—and sauntered off to the gift shop. Here, I'd also tried fry bread for the first time.

I was too late to have met Juan "Chief" Yellow Horse, a Diné native of Arizona who had come back from service as a Navy aviator in Berlin to take over a tourist attraction that had long occupied this lucrative corner between the Navajo lands on the north and the Petrified Forest on the south. Juan Yellow Horse, the subject of many travelers' snapshots in his eagle-feather headdress, died in 1999.

Today his son Scott Yellowhorse runs the shop. It's closing time, and he takes a break from turning a wrench underneath the hood of his truck to show us around. The trading post is filled with curiosities of all kinds; one can purchase the same array of refrigerator magnets and metal 66 shield cutouts as elsewhere, but there's much more to interest me: faded photographs of visitors past, a large assortment of secondhand books, bins of tumbled stones, well-made clothing and jewelry. A bit of cash changes hands. I ask Yellowhorse about the bison.

These days, he says, it's the dinosaurs—brightly colored statues—that get the kids' attention instead. We wave good-bye, let him get back to the car he's repairing, and move back out on the shadowed lanes of concrete.

Here, twenty-one years ago as an Easterner, I spied my first-ever live bison.

By Joseph City it's solid dark. With the guidance of a nearly-full moon we find the exit for a famous stretch of original Route 66 that long hosted roadhouses and rest stops for thirsty tourists. Back in the day entrepreneur James Taylor made his gift shop and desert museum unmissable across the country for those driving west, with a giant jackrabbit statue—complete with saddle for a photo op—and yellow-and-black mileage signs bearing the rabbit's silhouette and the slogan "HERE IT IS."

Real-life rabbits scurry from the beam of our headlights, which illuminate a closed-up shop, eerie in a parking lot seemingly populated by sleeping vehicles. Yep, too late. Well, There It Was.

We motor on to Winslow—where we compare the nightlife of the desert city to the daytime throngs accustomed to pulling over for another well-known photo op, "Standin' on the Corner." Even after restaurant-closing time, late arrivers like us pull in, read a bit of history, snap a selfie, spend a few dollars at the convenience store to refill our sodas. Who knew such innocuous opening lyrics would inspire the revitalization of an entire town? The city built its public park in 1999. It's estimated that each year some 100,000 visitors stop there these days. The Eagles themselves get a nod in the mural overlooking the permanently stationed flatbed Ford and the bronze statue of an unnamed guitarist (a separate figure depicts band member Glenn Frey).

It's worth the time to take it easy in Winslow, wander around and pick out all the cues from the song and the many public art installations that have followed from that first work.

After a layover in Flagstaff to write and publish the week's newspaper issues, we're refreshed and ready to take on one of the most challenging stretches of our journey.

I'd been reading blogs for weeks to keep up with road conditions and weather at Sitgreaves Pass, the high-elevation gateway to the old mining town of Oatman. While some Route 66 travelers—especially inexperienced motorcyclists—skip this winding, steep, unguardrailed segment, on a sunny summer morning it seems all systems go for our reliable pickup.

A swim and a good night's rest under neon lights in Kingman, an oil change, and a fortuitous tire check (removing three nails from our treads) make for a promising start. It's a good thing we've headed out early, as temperatures on the downslope would prove.

The climb up into the pass doesn't seem that daunting, at first; the narrow pavement's fine, the lane stripes brightly marked. But the switchbacks gradually slant steeper, the curves go blinder.

And then, the burros.

These are the primary hazard to bikers looking to keep up speed on the upslopes or harnessing it on the downside. The burros are the proliferant offspring of miners' beasts of burden turned loose once the minerals played out. Oatman became a ghost town in the 1940s, but the four-footed residents remained—and replicated. Today burros outnumber the human population five to one, except, of course, when tourists pour in, like today.

When a baby burro begs a bit of refreshment, or a herd ambles down

While some Route 66 travelers—especially inexperienced motorcyclists—skip this challenging, unguardrailed segment, on a sunny summer morning it seems all systems go for our reliable pickup.

the center line, vehicle traffic comes to a standstill. Oliver, leader of the pack, takes his sweet time, and his four-footed family ambles along behind. The two-wheeled and four-wheeled denizens of the Mother Road just have to bide their time.

The U.S. Bureau of Land Management conducts periodic roundups in the nearby desert by helicopter, relocating a few dozen burros at a time, according an AZCentral.com news piece earlier that year. "Burros have no natural predators, and I've watched them eat trees down to the ground," said John Hall, who manages BLM's wild horse and burro program in Arizona.

But the burros without doubt keep old Oatman alive with travelers, in an obviously symbiotic relationship. As temperatures approach their 116-degree high today, the human occupants of Oatman flock to the numerous watering holes, old-fashioned photo booths and T-shirt shops to leave a few bucks behind.

Would we have regretted bypassing this chapter in our westward travels? You bet your sweet Sitgreaves Pass we would. ☞

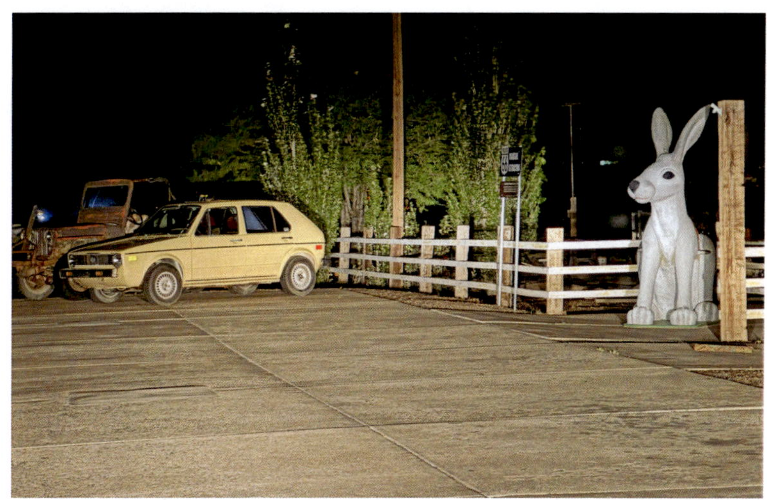

RABBITS OF DIFFERENT SORTS have multiplied at the Jack Rabbit Route 66 gift shop in Joseph City, Arizona. A scary-looking giant rabbit—saddled up for photo ops—was replaced some years ago with this happier one, and was joined by a yellow VW Rabbit on the site.

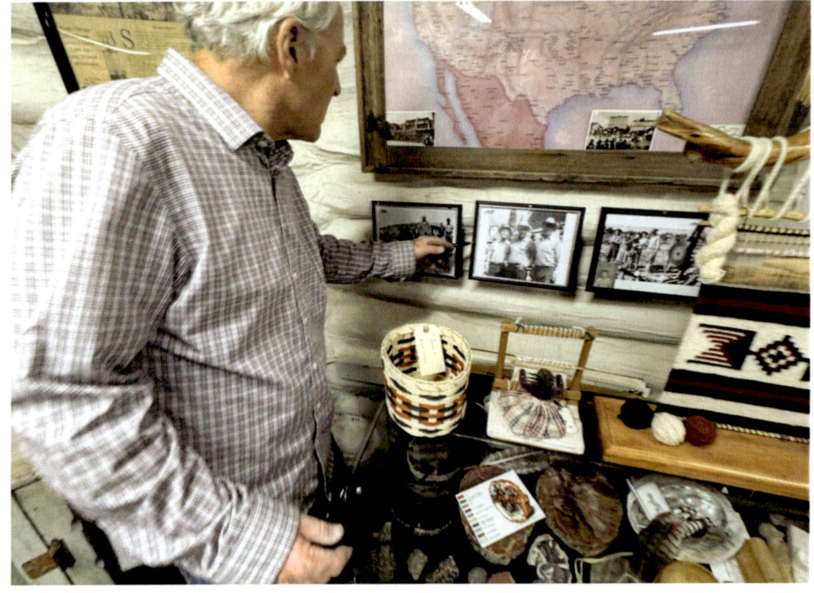

SCOTT YELLOWHORSE continues his family tradition of welcoming tourists along Route 66/I-40 at the New Mexico–Arizona state line.

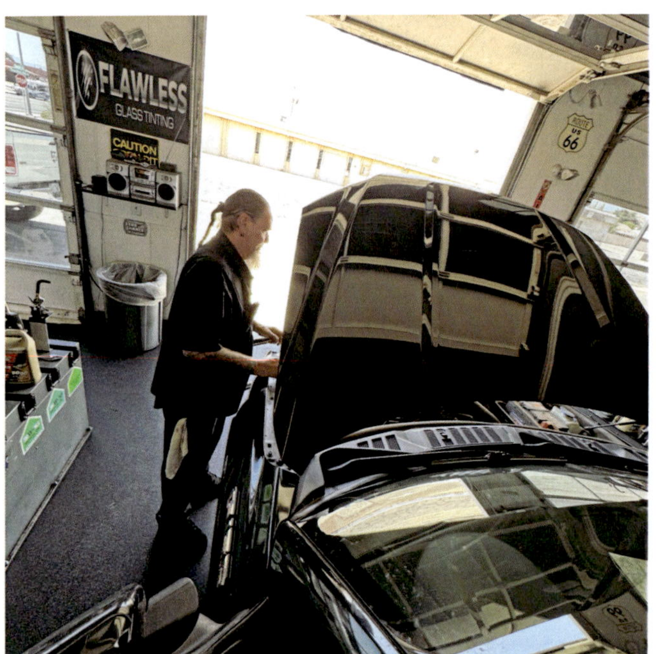

BLACK BEAUTY, our intrepid F-150, gets a much-needed wash, oil change, and tire service at a friendly shop in Kingman, Arizona.

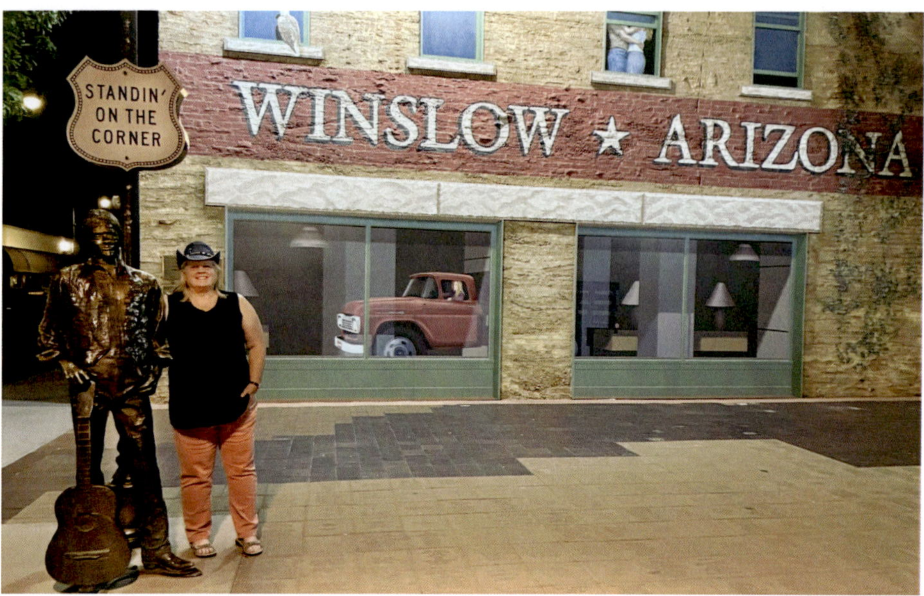

TAKE IT EASY Twenty-one years (and maybe even more pounds) after my first visit to Winslow, I renewed may acquaintance with the unnamed guitarist depicted in the Eagles tribute. Jackson Browne (never officially a member of the Eagles) started the work on "Take it Easy," the band's 1972 first hit, but was stuck on the second verse. Glenn Frey added the famous "flatbed Ford" line, and Browne gifted the song to the band.

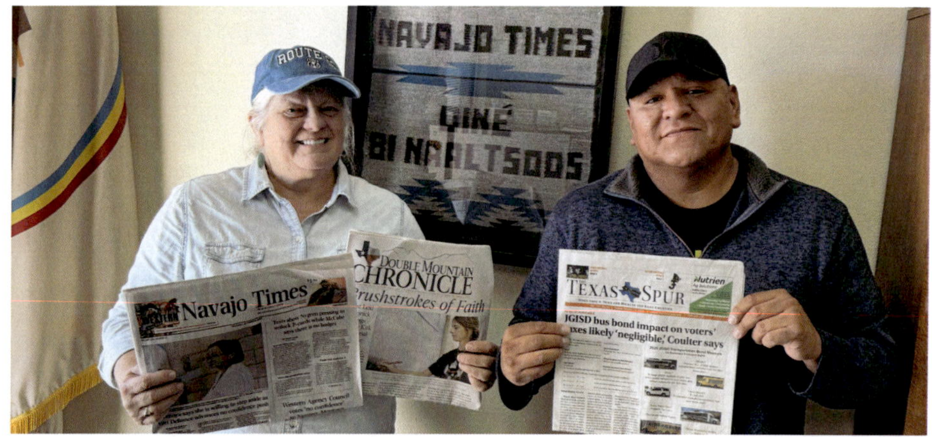

NEWSPAPER SWAP The Navajo Times is the largest independent, Native American-owned weekly newspaper in the U.S., based in Window Rock, Arizona, capital of the Navajo Nation. Founded in 1959 as a tribal newsletter, today it counts a circulation of 24,900 with more than 150,000 weekly readers. Our Texas Spur staff dropped by the paper's offices in October 2025.

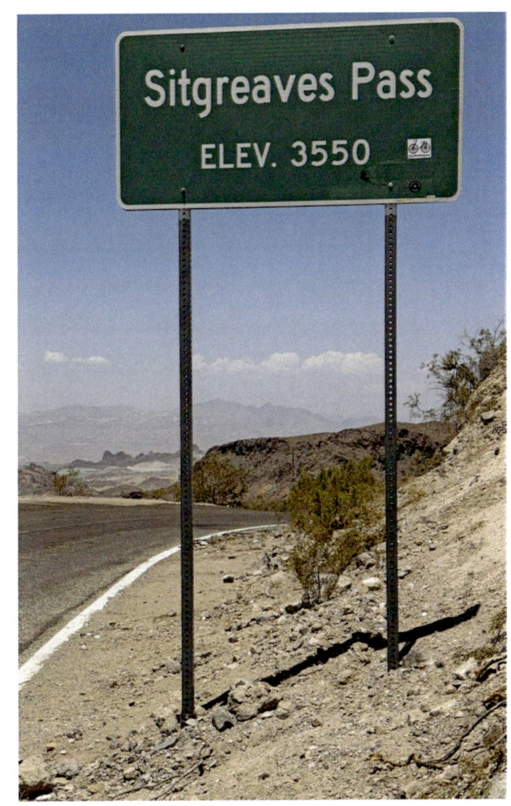

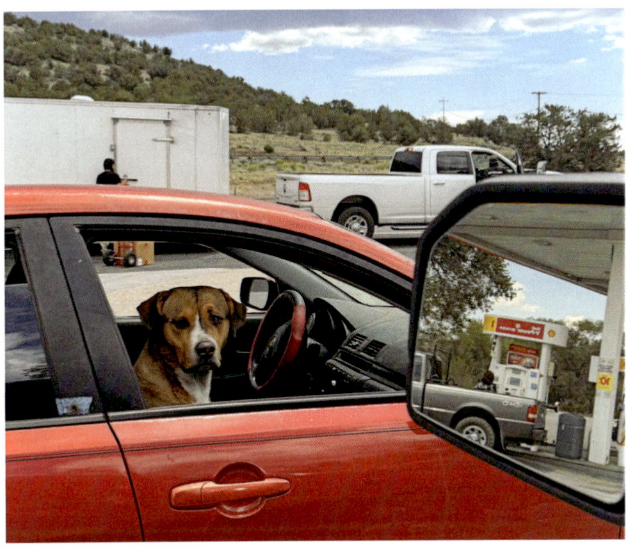

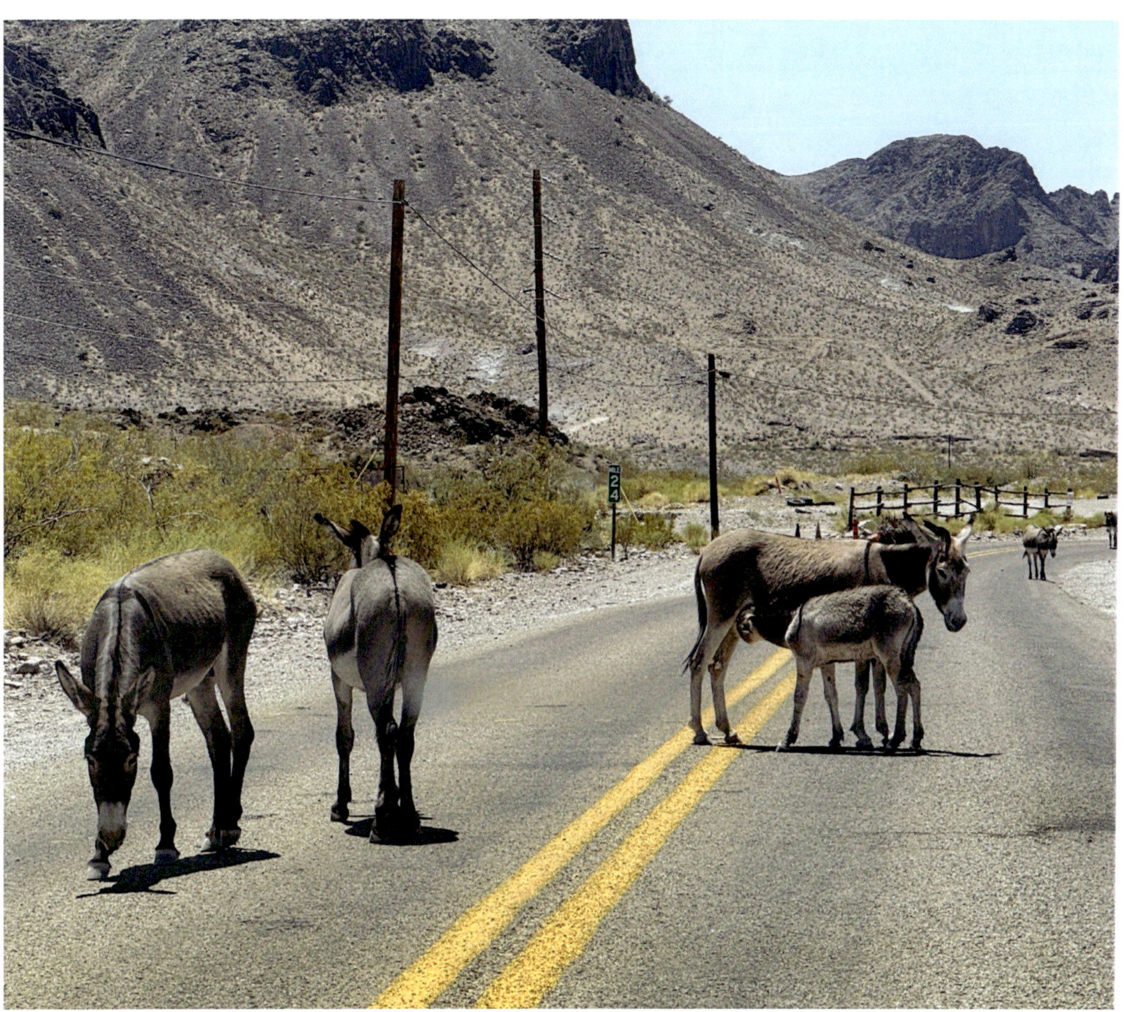

BURROS RULE THE ROAD in this high-elevation stretch of the Mother Road (especially the mother burros)—and drivers must exercise caution!

DON'T FORGET WINONA At the small Route 66 town east of Flagstaff, Arizona, this pooch looks ready to motor west.

CHAPTER EIGHT

California dreamin' and driving

IN THE AMERICAN CONSCIOUSNESS, California occupies a fabled throne: lodestone of the Golden West, goal of the beleaguered Dust Bowl Okies, fantasy of film and fortune, home of the high life.

The part of this vast state you'll experience along the remnants of Route 66 provides fleeting views of all this and more. Yet between the glittering glimpses lie miles of baking desert and miles of multilane concrete, neither of which is avoidable on the journey to Nirvana. Perhaps there are better times to make that journey than the hottest July on record.

Still, the blue Pacific waters beckon, and even the desert has its special fascinations.

Among those, the stretch of the Mother Road known as the National Old Trails Highway west of Needles proved challenging in some ways, soothing in others. With no reservation and no particular destination other than the inevitable End of the Trail, we were in the perfect situation to observe this 130 miles of old blacktop: unhurried, plenty of gas in the tank purchased at Arizona prices, iced-down beverages, and a superbly functioning air conditioning system. We had it way better than the Joads.

The road veers south of I-40 on a trajectory that follows an old railroad route between the Mojave National Preserve on the north and the Sheephole

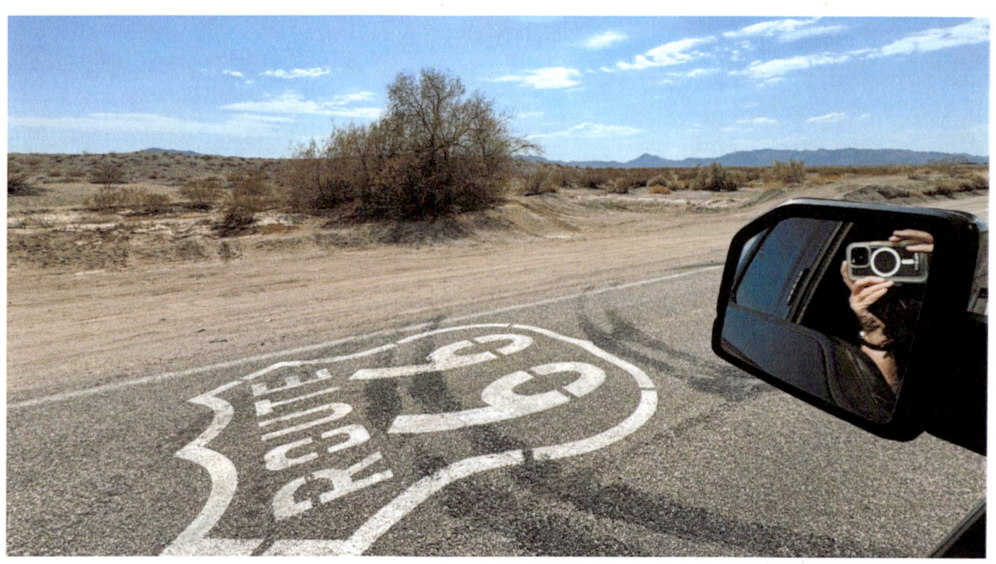

THE ROAD TO AMBOY beckons with the Route 66 shield painted on the pavement and the mountain range across the desert in the distance.

Once over the San Gabriel mountains and into San Bernardino, I found the drive reminiscent of watching an old home movie, with what used to be distinct, individual towns rolling by in fluid sequence.

Valley and Cleghorn Lakes Wilderness areas to the south. In reverse alpha order we cruise past former train stops: Essex, Danby, Chambless. We've passed no vehicles coming from the west; and only one other from the east, a red convertible that quickly overtook our pace and disappeared over the hazy late-afternoon horizon. At our leisurely speed it's easy to spot the humanmade intrusions into the landscape: a monument to Route 66; an group of low-slung, abandoned buildings; a pair of bleached-marble Chinese lions, standing watch in the distance.

At the ghost town of Amboy, pop. zero according to a recent feature in *The Los Angeles Times,* the futuristic angles of the Roy's Café sign are even more unmissable. The ultimate monument to the traffic-siphoning effect of I-40, the former wayside store, service station, and motel complex, shuttered in 1972.

Southern California businessman Albert Okura, "The Chicken Man with a 50 Year Plan" that once included moving the corporate headquarters of

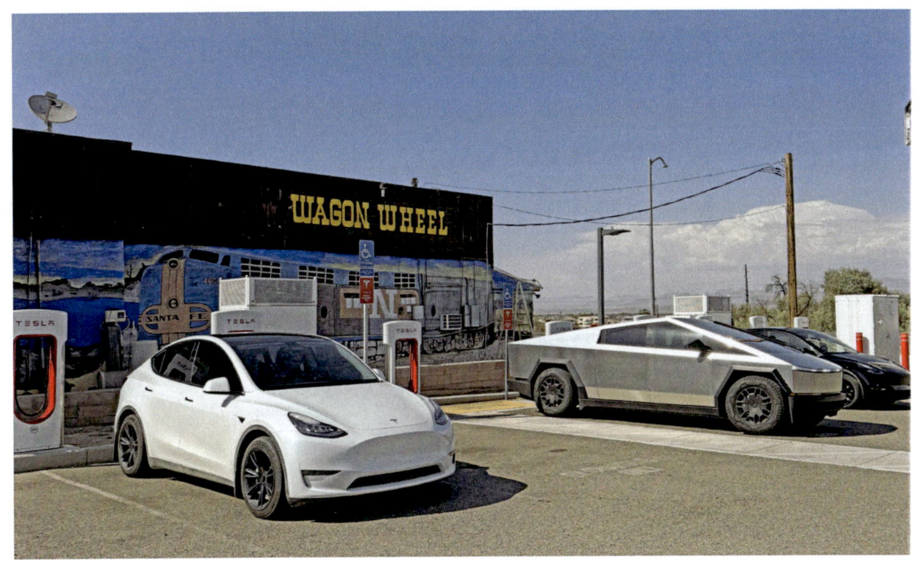

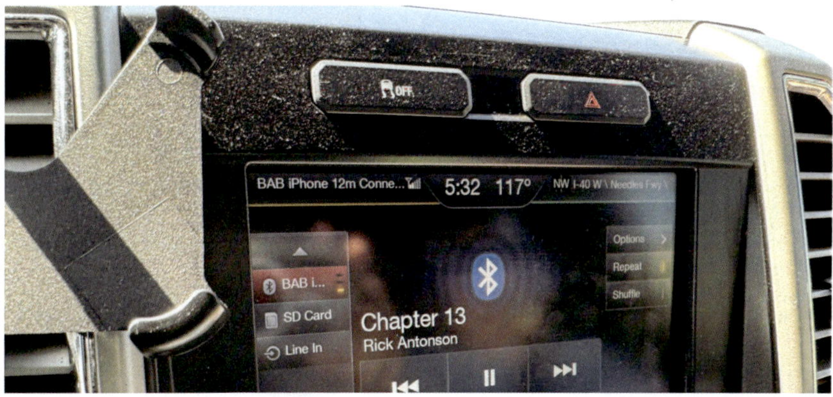

TOPOCK TEMP topped 117 as we crossed from arid Arizona into scorching California—a state that took its name from a 16th-century Spanish romance that described a mythical island paradise. In July 2024, the hottest ever since official meteorological records began in 1895, it was no paradise.

IN NEEDLES, CALIFORNIA the local convenience store harks back to a much earlier mode of travel—while empowering newer ones. All along the Route, but especially in California, we spotted plenty of Tesla electric Cybertrucks.

his Juan Pollo restaurant chain into the original McDonald's building in San Bernardino, bought Amboy in 2005. The whole town. He restored gas service and a snack bar, amenities that continue to serve travelers under the operation of his son, Kyle. The senior Okura saw revitalization of the town as his destiny; his son carries on that legacy today.

But as in so many places along the Route, we've arrived too late to benefit from local commerce. We enjoy our photo session alone, two kids in the amusement park after the gates have been shut.

Overnighting in Victorville gives us a chance to cleanse away the desert dust in a lovely swimming pool once the evening temps have dipped down into the 90s. We repack in anticipation of the homeward journey that will commence in a couple of days.

We refresh our maps, preparing to follow the thread of original 66 routing amid the tangle of Los Angeles freeways. This turned out to be not as hard as we'd feared over the past 2,400 miles; it would simply take some patience with traffic, and the willingness to backtrack and reconnect when a turn had been missed. Swift glimpses of California icons were our reward.

Once over the San Gabriel mountains and into San Bernardino, I found the drive reminiscent of watching an old home movie, with what used to be distinct, individual towns rolling by in fluid sequence: Rancho Cucamonga, Pasadena, Glendale. Before long we reached place-names that were even more deeply etched in the memory of show and song: Sunset Boulevard, Hollywood Hills, Santa Monica Boulevard. The Troubador. We paused our extended film reel only to detour for stills (to Dodgers Stadium, for instance, or the Hollywood sign, or the Capitol Records Tower).

In this way we surely overlooked some of the most legendary Route 66 roadside attractions we'd been learning about via podcast; but oddly we gained a more seamless appreciation for the road itself. Not its younger, slicked-back, saucier self ever in search of the next adventure, but its more seasoned, laid-back, twenty-first-century persona, angles and edges smoothed over, ripe with experience, welcoming the traveler with every modern convenience. As city melts into city, from West Hollywood to Beverly Hills to Century City to Santa Monica, the road becomes a composite of our entire 2024 experience: more homogenized, branded, packaged. Not even the stop-and-go traffic fazes us; we are in our bubble, floating along the asphalt river.

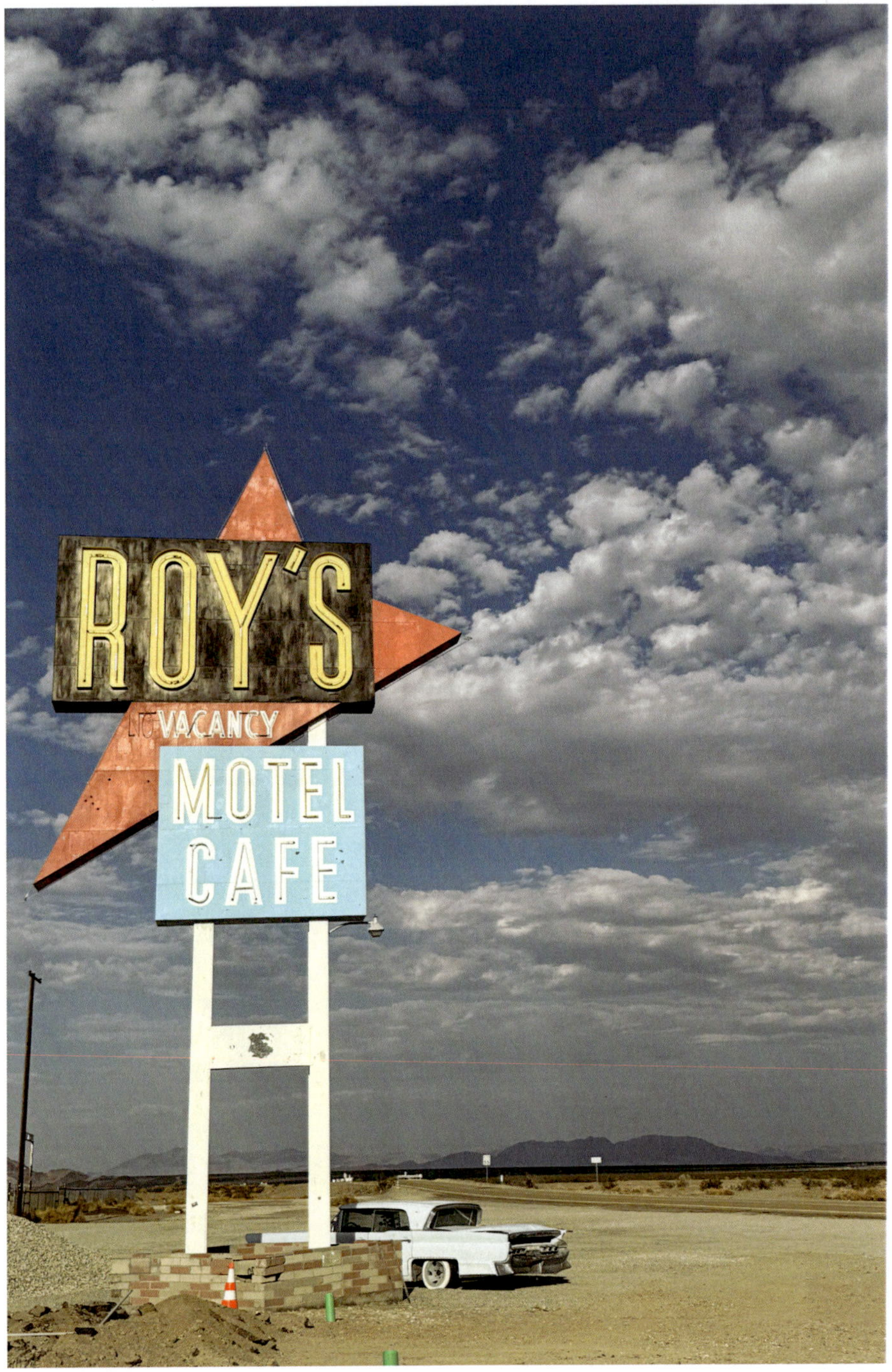

ROY CROWL built a complex of tourist services along Route 66 in Amboy in the 1940s, but in 1972 the coming of I-40 a few miles to the north left his enterprises cut off. The day we breezed through, gas (which must be pumped by an attendant during open hours) was going for $6.49 a gallon.

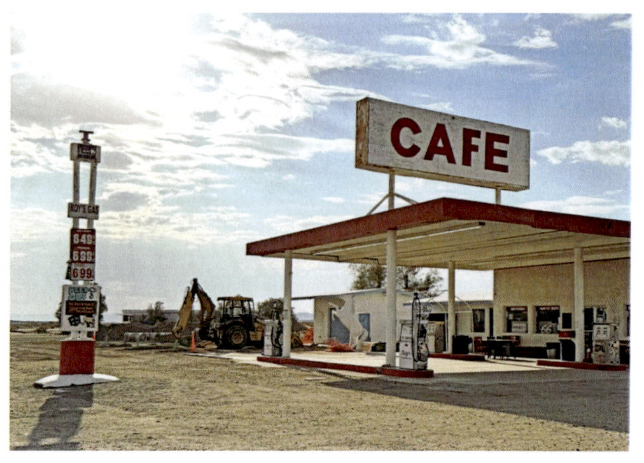

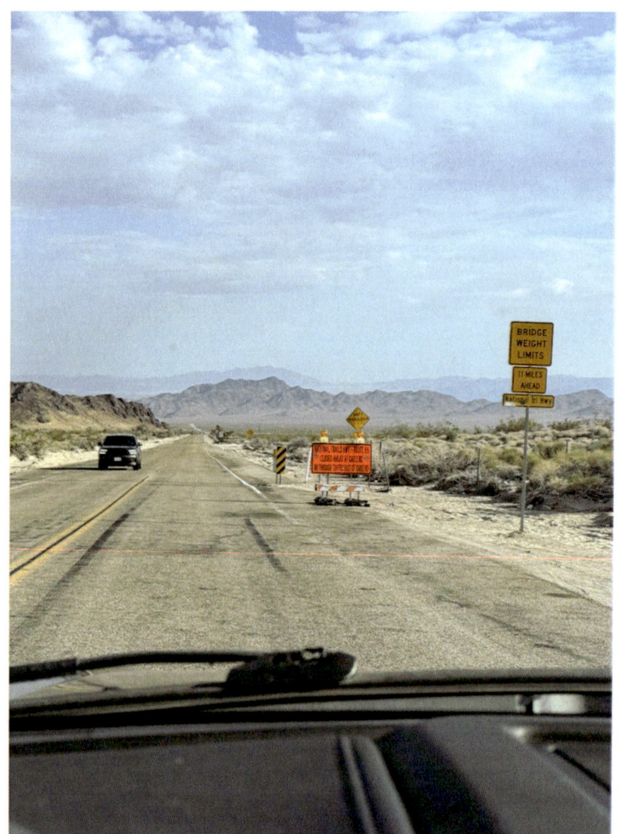

ROAD CLOSED In the Southern California deserts, many two-lane roads—including surviving stretches of Route 66—were badly damaged by tropical storm washouts in recent decades and have remained unrepaired.

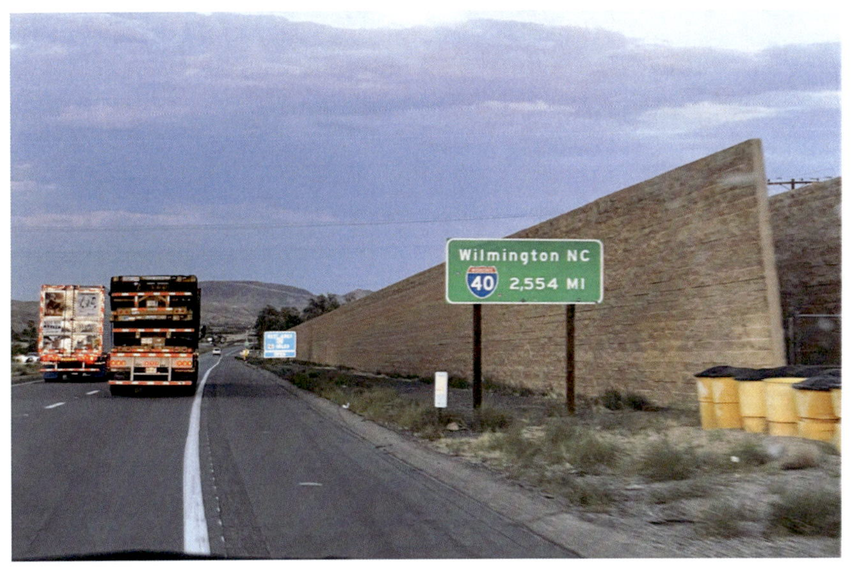

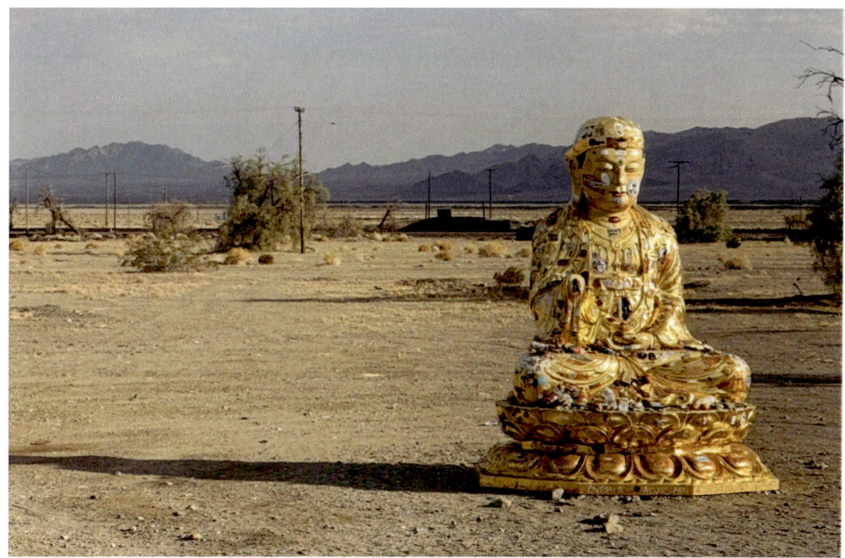

WILMINGTON NC 2,554 MI is the flip side of a similar green Interstate sign located near the eastbound terminus of I-40. Twenty-one years ago I traveled here from Wilmington, pulled off on the shoulder here and took one of my first selfies ever, underneath this very sign (flip back to page 5 if you missed it).

BUDDHA IN THE DESERT is one of the mysteries along this isolated stretch of the Mother Road.

AMID LOS ANGELES TRAFFIC Scott Froschauer's 2020 public-art installation (far right) provides a suitable sentiment.

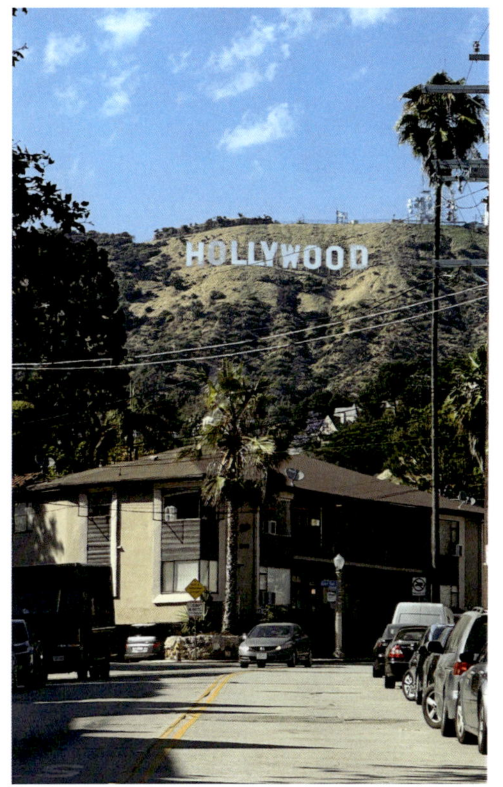

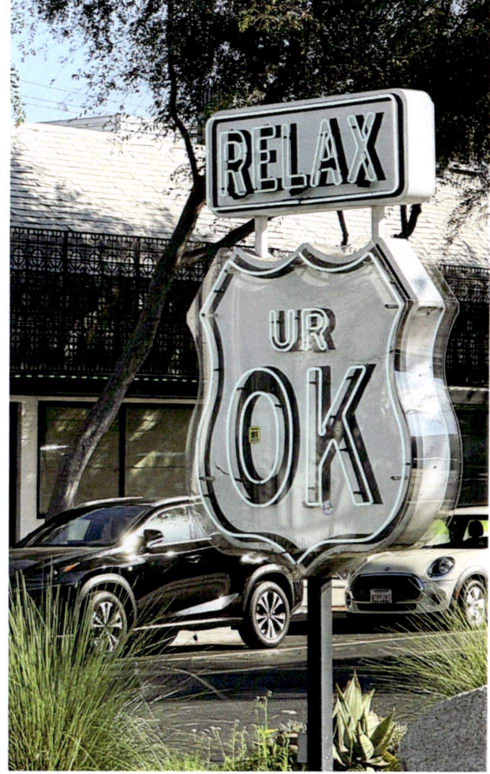

MID-CENTURY MODERN and "Googie"-style architecture are a treat all along Route 66, especially at cafes and gas stations. This one (left) is in Hesperia, California.

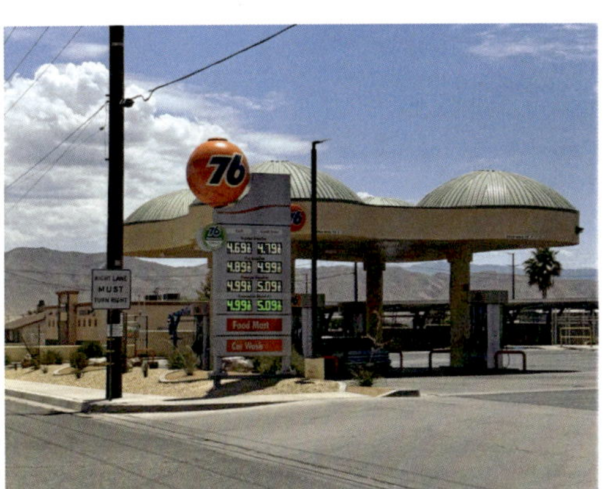

So many of the logos visible along this storied road are
the same we've seen back home—and many originated here
or are based here. Netflix, Tesla, Blockbuster, McDonald's.
This phenomenon itself is part of the story of America. To
find the outliers, the unconventional, the "authentic" we
so seek may take some work. And maybe it's not exactly
"original" we're looking for after all; it's hard to get more
inventive than the McDonald brothers, or Elon Musk. It's
the spark of something individual and imaginative, perhaps,
that still stands out in only one place.

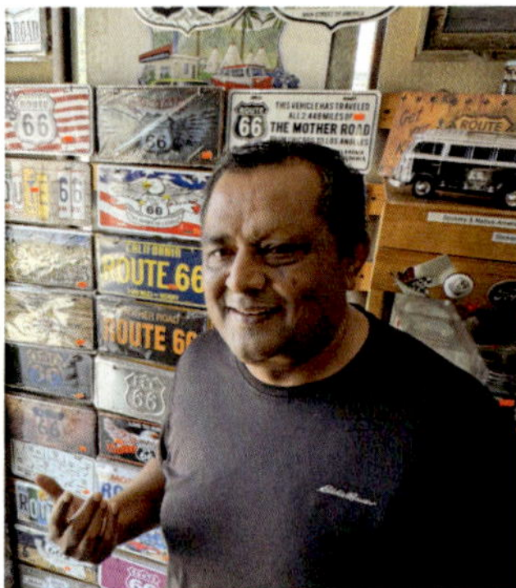

Read enough of the roadies' blogs, and you'll be reminded that Route 66 reached its
western terminus at the intersection of Lincoln and Olympic in Santa Monica. In the early-
evening crowds we cruise by that landmark in a blink of an eye, not realizing till half a mile
onward that we'd swept right past the photo op.

 But at the Santa Monica Pier, long a magnet for fishing, fun and film scouts, it's far
easier to park your car, stretch your legs, and indulge your appetite. For date night or
family outing, the pier is a mini-amusement park complete with Ferris wheel and carnival
vendors, sit-down restaurants and hot-dog stands, informational displays and photo ops.

Route 66 roadie Dan Rice of Los Angeles recognized the perfect opportunity back in
2009, when Mother Road tourism was beginning to take off again. "How could there be
nothing to mark the end of the most famous road in the world?" he wrote on his website,
66toCali.com.

So he made one. That year he created an "End of the Trail" marker and installed it on
the pier alongside his souvenir shop specializing in made-in-the-USA T-shirts. A legend
was born. The legend was cultivated with 66toCali's Certificate of Completion, which
visitors can also obtain at the shop.

On that final evening of our journey, shop manager Ian Bowen welcomed us Texans
and happily signed our certificates. We stood in line behind crowds waiting to pony up
for those T-shirts, hoodies, mugs, and magnets, too. Money changed hands, food was

SLEEP IN A TEEPEE — it's still possible at the clean, well-run Wigwam Motel in Rialto (San Berdardino), California,
where generations of travelers have delighted in the kitschy, if inaccurately named, design. In 1933, wrote the current
owners on their website, Frank Redford first started developing the Wigwam "Villages" by designing tipi-shaped
motel units around a museum-cum-shop he had built to showcase his Native American artifacts. He went on to build
seven motels using his wigwam design; the one in San Bernardino was his last.

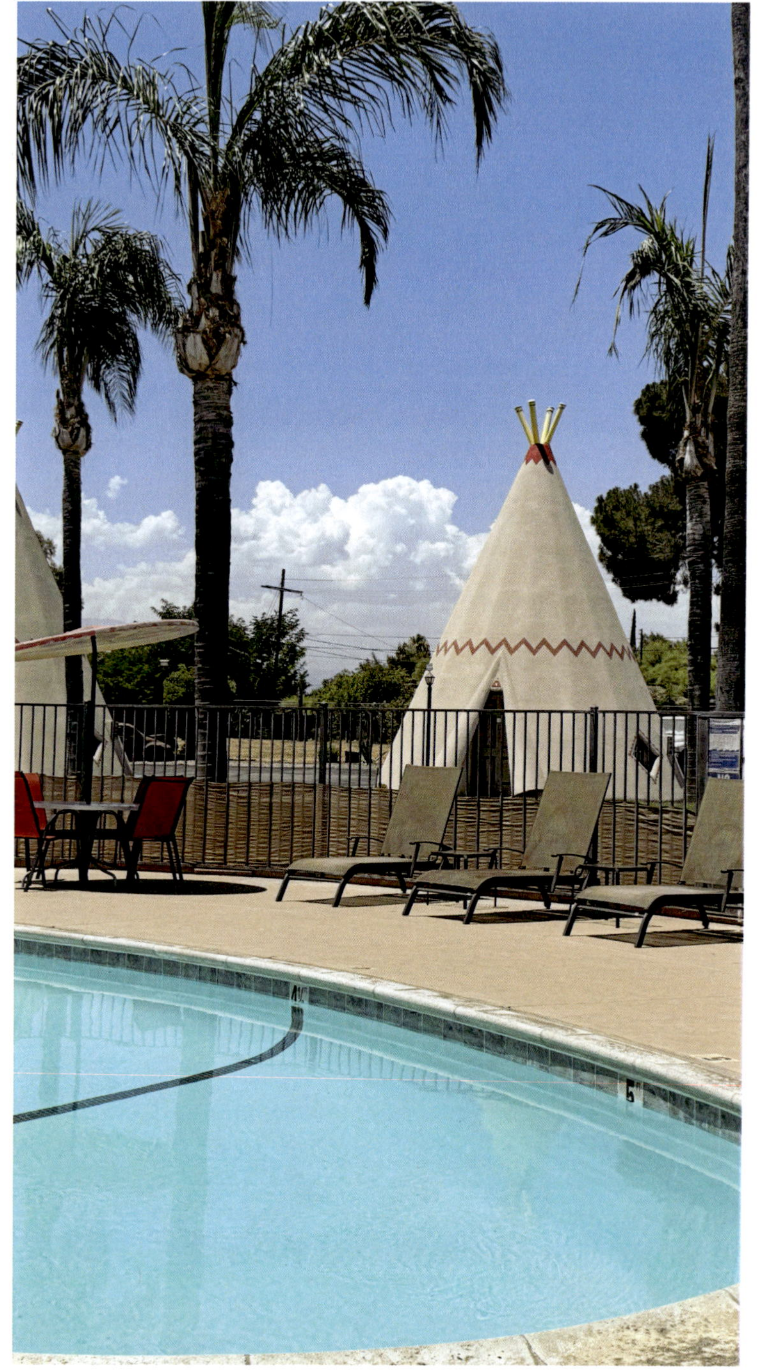

consumed, selfies were taken. People had a great time, the surf rolled beneath us as the sun set over the Pacific on a pleasant evening of leisure and love for some, commerce and creativity for others. Now, if that isn't American ingenuity, what is?

Driving back to our lodgings for the night, a concrete teepee in Rialto where third-generation Asian immigrants still run the family business, we heartily agree.

We settle into our folding camp chairs in the parking lot to watch the moon rise over the palms. The gentlest of breezes masks the occasional sounds along the road outside our motel door: engines revving, conversations among pedestrians, a police siren, a barking dog. The surface of the blue pool ripples.

A beverage from the cooler is our toast to the Mother Road.

Long may she flourish, as she approaches her milestone birthday.

Tomorrow, we'll start making our plans to celebrate it. ☞

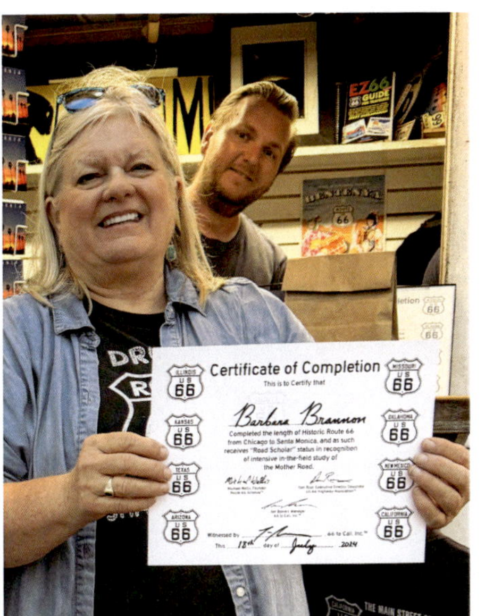

66toCALI at the T-shirt stand on the Santa Monica Pier, merchant and artist Ian Bowen presented us our Route 66 Certificates of Completion.

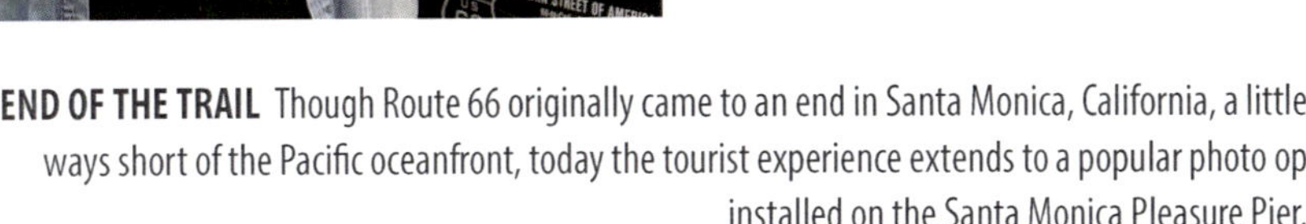

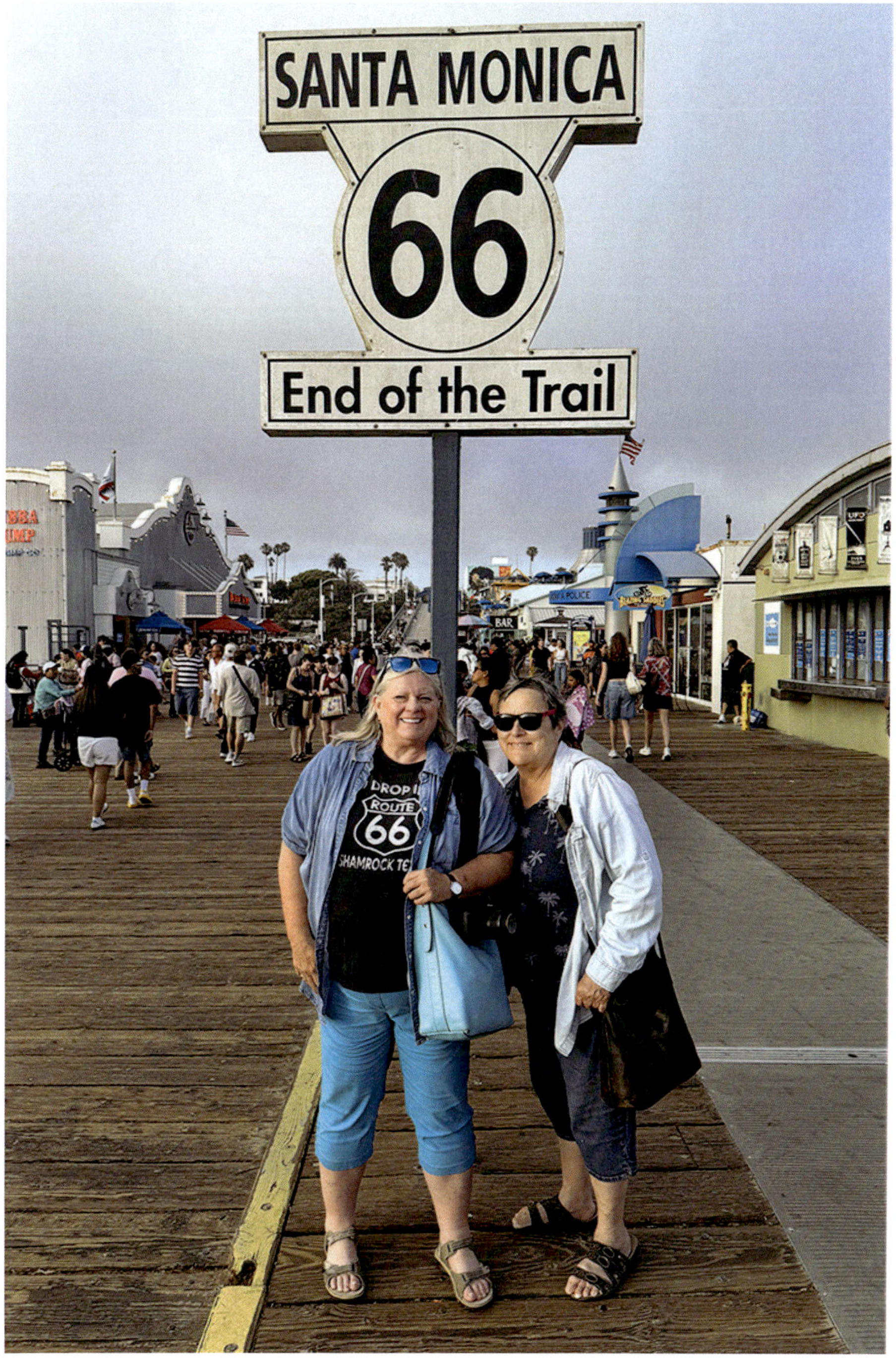

END OF THE TRAIL Though Route 66 originally came to an end in Santa Monica, California, a little ways short of the Pacific oceanfront, today the tourist experience extends to a popular photo op installed on the Santa Monica Pleasure Pier.

CHAPTER NINE

Home to Texas— with Mother Road memories

We're often prompted by leisure-travel marketers to think of our journeys as "making memories," and this must indeed be a strong urge for families planning vacations, couples designing destination weddings, school groups deciding where to go for the senior class trip.

But for my money the most valuable aspects of the Route 66 drive are the musings to come. What does our past, experienced and considered in the present, signal about our future as a nation? Such ideas can be cultivated piecemeal, of course, over years; our summer 2024 trip was layered onto the cross-country drive in 2003 that had incorporated much of Route 66, and many, many day trips to states like Oklahoma and New Mexico in between. Rambles later in 2024 and 2025 added richness and complexity to our experience.

The singular opportunity for one continuous drive at an unhurried pace is like reading a novel—or,

Thank you for sticking with us from Texas to Chicago to Los Angeles and back. We welcome your feedback, and your own memories, at Facebook/Route66Ramble

maybe more accurately, a volume of history—from cover to cover, rather than picking up a collection of short stories and dipping in from time to time. Or like watching a film in a theater rather than sitting down in front of the TV for an hour-long drama once a week.

The result is a panorama of the westering urge that helps to place the centuries of American migration into some perspective. From the arrival of newcomers on the continent's shores with a sense of wonder and conquest, to the continual pushing-out of indigenous inhabitants from their homelands into ever more arid landscapes, to the establishment of industry and agriculture across the continent, the story unfolds in one extended sitting.

It isn't always a noble history. On our cross-country rambles we traversed locations where slave or migrant labor built the rails and later the roads, cultivated the fields, worked in the lodgings and eateries—or were often refused service in them.

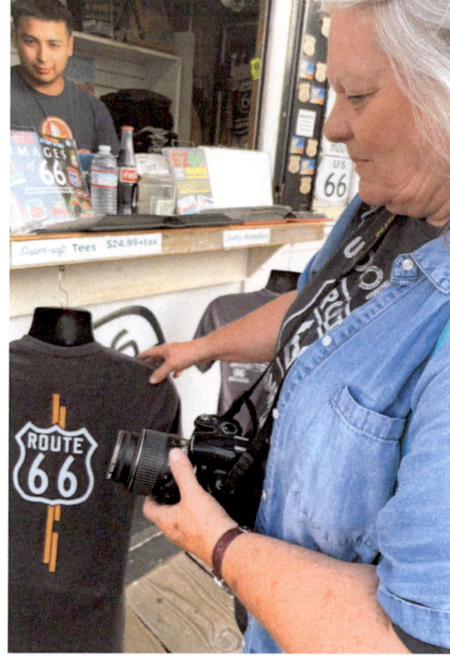

DROVE THE 2,448 MILES, GOT THE T-SHIRT
Braggin' rights and a signed souvenir "certificate of completion" are fun to keep in the memory box, along with hundreds of travel brochures, a replica keychain to a wigwam motel, and a few new books for the sagging bookshelf. Thanks for riding along on our journey! For more (many, many more) photos, visit www.flickr.com/photos/barbarabrannon

We've seen blight, urban sprawl, decay, crime, poverty, greed. (One need only contrast the multitudes of roofless sleepers along Albuquerque's sidewalks against the thousands of lightbulbs beckoning gamblers' wallets to the nearby casino.)

But it is a living one. If we're all coming "to look for America," no matter who we are, from this country or outside it, we'll find something of ourselves along the Mother Road. The two-lane generously gives back our respect for it, and all our efforts to protect it will be rewarded for generations to come.

All along the Route, from Illinois to California, the people we met were friendly, interesting and helpful. From Bill Thomas in Atlanta, Illinois, who helped us gain perspective on The Road Ahead, to Donna in Joplin, to Brenda in Adrian, to the tire guy in Kingman, to the Patels in San Bernardino, our way was made smooth by those who've gone before us.

It didn't take long, after pulling into the driveway in Spur once more, to unpack suitcases, dump the cooler, and pick the bugs from the radiator grille. It didn't take long to settle back into the regular seven-day cycle of news coverage, or the habits of householding. But I knew we'd be spending long months unpacking observations recorded in a handful of journals, processing photos and uploading them (www.flickr.com/photos/barbarabrannon), and putting down these pages an extended record of the journey.

The ten-week series of essays in *The Texas Spur* and our other weekly newspapers were a good start on that. We appreciate the readers who stuck with us from Texas to Chicago to Los Angeles and back.

May your own journeys always be as fruitful as this one was for us. Stay safe, make friends, and keep your camera and journal always ready. ☞

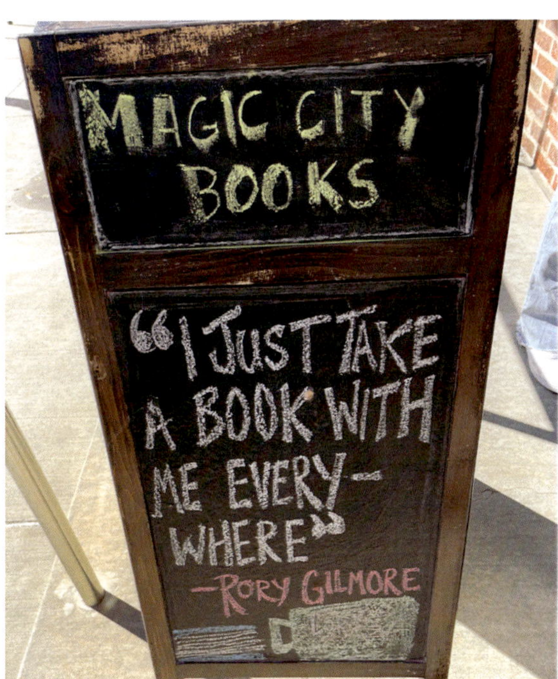

INDIE BOOKSTORE Magic City Books of Tulsa, Oklahoma, has the right idea for life—and travel.

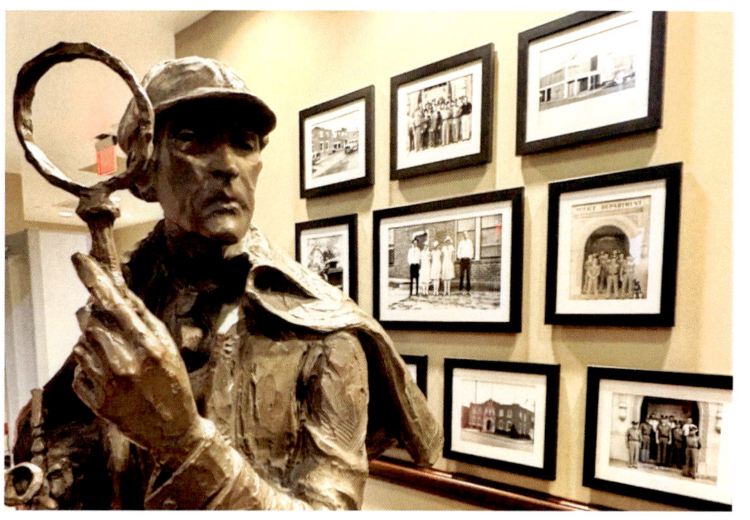

HOLMES ON THE ROUTE Conan Doyle's intrepid detective Sherlock Holmes may have tracked more bicycles and Victorian hackneys than motor cars—but a larger-than-life bronze inside the Edmond, Oklahoma, police department, a block off Old Route 66, pays tribute to his methods and reminds us all to keep our eyes open for the telling detail. (Ask us about why we experienced the inside of the Edmond PD on a rainy summer morning. That's a whole other adventure.)

HESPERIA HIGH SCHOOL—"Home of the Scorpions" in the California desert— pays tribute to the westward inclination that also gives us the word "vespers."

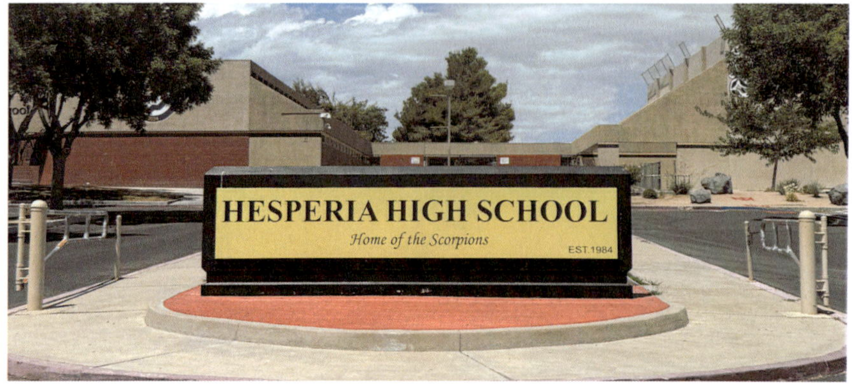

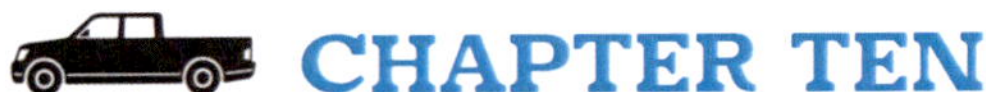 **CHAPTER TEN**

This Land Is Your Land

This land is your land, this land is my land.

But is it, really, after the divisions our nation has experienced since January 6, 2021, or November 5, 2024, or events of fall 2025 in the city of Minneapolis? How shall we then live, as Americans, or in America?

Some months after returning from our summer 2024 Route 66 through-drive, Kay and I posed these questions to a community gathering in our home state in observance of Veterans Day in November 2024, also the week following a contentious presidential election.

Writers long before us, from Katherine Lee Bates to Woody Guthrie to John Steinbeck, Robert Pirsig to William Least Heat-Moon, from Martin Luther King, Jr., to Cheryl Strayed to Jessica Bruder to Tim Z. Hernandez, have likewise asked this question of us and themselves. Numerous thinkers have challenged our country's dominant, default position of privilege. Steinbeck, in particular, hit the road during a troubling season in the nation's evolution characterized by racial strife and a loss of authenticity in the early 1960s.

We have traveled together across many states and countries, we told those gathered in a safe space among friends. We had driven the country to see what made us tick, and to join in a dialogue about what we'd witnessed.

We've hiked together, camped together, and ridden many, many ferries together, we said. But on our 2024 journey we had a particular objective in mind, as our country's iconic Route 66 approached its hundredth anniversary and I experienced my own 66th year. We were back later that year, and since.

While the Mother Road doesn't stretch quite from sea to shining sea, its reach from Navy Pier in Chicago, Illinois, to Santa Monica Pier in California embraces landmarks as storied as Lake Michigan and the Pacific Ocean; the mighty Mississippi River and the mesas of New Mexico; Texas plains and Arizona mountain passes; drive-ins, deserts, neon lights. Its cities are legendary, its small towns fascinating, its skies wide, its people diverse.

The week before our Route 66 trip, presidential candidates had faced off in an unsatisfying debate. The uncertainties of that event left many citizens anxious about our nation's future—by now, of course, our present reality.

But we weren't there yet, when Kay and I set out on our Route 66 journey. Our sense of expectation rode high, and anticipation fueled the many miles of travel that lay ahead. If we had a defined goal, it was to drive all of the storied highway in one continuous trip, to grasp as much as humanly possible of what unifies and defines "the Route 66 experience." To see it like a long movie with fascinating characters, in one uninterrupted theater sitting.

This book—as the talk we gave that day—presents a few clips from our movie.

Our journey didn't lack for iconic photo ops, or amusing Muffler Men, or Cosmic Travelers, or Giant Women, or the homes of presidents, we observed. But it was in Abraham Lincoln's presidential library, in Springfield, Illinois, that we came face to face with the reality that acrimony was nothing new in our nation's public sphere.

Down the road in Joplin, Missouri, public art works frequently treated themes of healing from intolerance of others, a topic we would see repeated in Tulsa, Oklahoma—once the scene of devastating race riots—or in sites like Miami, Oklahoma, where Native American heritage was proudly claimed, or among pueblo communities in the desert Southwest, or in the culturally, ethnically, and gender-diverse neighborhoods of greater Los Angeles.

Ideological statements took many clever forms. Not all were as boldly emblazoned as Woody Guthrie's scrawled words "This Machine Kills Fascists" on the body of his guitar.

At the historic Rainbow Bridge in Kansas it was heartening and healing to encounter creative collaborators, a local photographer and a musician who put on a fundraising event for veterans.

All along the route we witnessed cycles of prosperity, decline, and rebirth—thanks to the unifying thread of the Mother Road. In the old mining town of Galena, Kansas, where we met Police Chief Billy Charles, the story of the animated movie *Cars* helped us see what was worth preserving across our landscape twenty years ago, and what was at risk of neglect and ruin.

We spent half a day on those 12 miles of Route 66 in Kansas before crossing into Oklahoma. We had begun to fully appreciate the revival brought about by one movie. "Cars" culture was everywhere. If Lightning McQueen had been the savior of Route 66, ushering in a whole new era of fame for the road, its prophet had been journalist Michael Wallis, author of the award-winning 1990 book *Route 66: The Mother Road*.

These days, Wallis is hardly a lone voice in the wilderness. Many fans and preservationists have joined in. Support—and dollars—have flowed. On the cusp of a nationwide Route 66 birthday party long in the making, we'll have a full year of events to pick from.

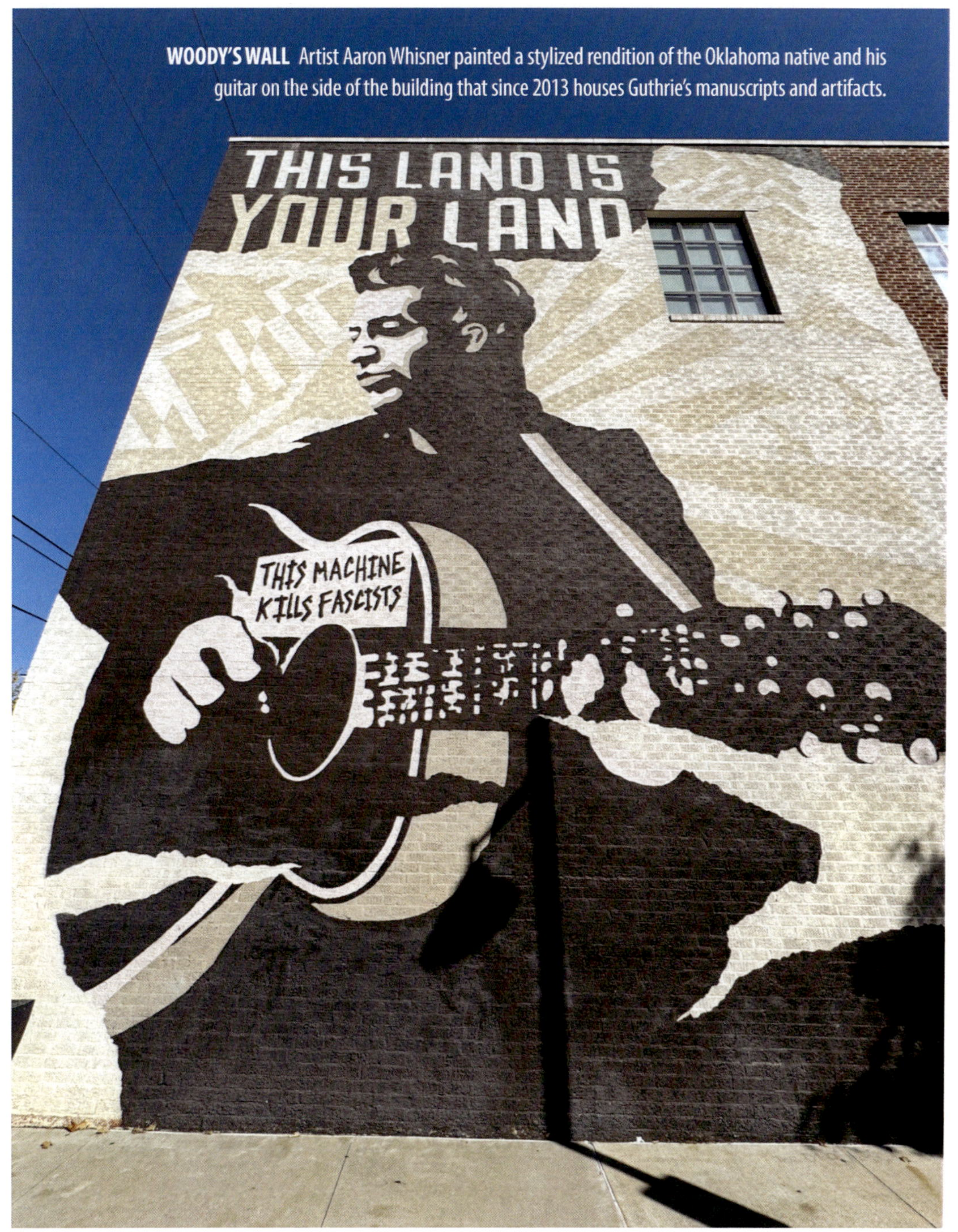

WOODY'S WALL Artist Aaron Whisner painted a stylized rendition of the Oklahoma native and his guitar on the side of the building that since 2013 houses Guthrie's manuscripts and artifacts.

In Oklahoma, where Route 66 makes its pronounced bend westward, we could sense our nation's diversity as we crossed counties named for Native tribes who had been forcibly resettled there, and as horses and cowboy hats became ubiquitous. It was also home to figures like baseball great Mickey Mantle, actor Alfre Woodard, country artist Garth Brooks, writer S. E. Hinton of *The Outsiders.* And of course the humorist and commentator Will Rogers, who often held forth on politics and loved to sling barbs at Democrats and Republicans alike.

A couple of them: "Party politics is the most narrow minded occupation in the World" and "Elections are a good deal like marriages, there's no accounting for anyone's taste."

Will Rogers had no idea.

Oklahoma also claims the longest stretch of Route 66 that is still accessible for driving today, according to Rhys Martin, a Tulsa native and director of his state's Route 66 preservation program.

Let's take a minute to review the history lesson. When the highway was first designated in 1926, thanks to roads advocate Cyrus Avery of Tulsa, it represented a whole new era of easier travel across America on uniform, federally maintained roadway. The individual states were tasked with surveying, mapping, surfacing, maintaining, signing.

Route 66 offered a way to cross a vast nation with better weather than other options. The National Park Service history of Route 66 notes that "many of the merchants in the small and large towns through which the highway passed looked to the road as an economic opportunity to bring much needed outside revenues into their often rural and isolated communities."

It took twelve years to get the whole 2,448 miles paved. By then, many Dust Bowl refugees and Hollywood opportunists had traversed parts of it to reach the golden West. The road gained mythic status thanks in part to John Steinbeck's 1939 novel *The Grapes of Wrath* then postwar popularity by 1946, when Nat King Cole recorded Bobby Troup's "Get Your Kicks on Route 66." Mom-and-pop motels, chain restaurants, vacation attractions flourished throughout the mid-century.

During this heyday of vacation road trips, it's worth noting how few

We all came here from somewhere. We all rode the same roads to get here. And where we're going, there will always have been others, who did, or didn't, look like us.

facilities courted, or catered to, the Black population; a decade ago Candacy Taylor's Route 66 Green Book Project research revealed that "according to the 1930 Census, 44 out of the 89 counties along Route 66 were all white." It's shocking to put this in context: "Even once travelers reached a multiracial city such as Albuquerque, their options were still limited," she wrote, with a miniscule proportion of available lodgings accepting Negro travelers. Even fewer such Route 66 properties listed in the Negro Green Book remain today.

By 1985, the entirety of Route 66, doomed by the high-speed Interstate system, deemed obsolete and decommissioned as a U.S. highway, was left unfunded and unsigned. For years now, stretches of the road have been left to the elements, cut off from access, or sealed over by Interstate concrete.

That nostalgia—popularized by the *Cars* movie—has fueled a renaissance today. A decade ago, the eight Route 66 states got serious about unified efforts to preserve what remained of The Mother Road.

In San Bernardino, California, our journey almost done, we talked with third-generation hotelier Kumar Patel. The visit helped put a few things in perspective.

Patel, whose family had bought the hotel in 2003 from the original owners, is a champion of Route 66 travel who loves to show off photos and artifacts in the motel's tiny lobby.

An Asian Indian operating a lodging establishment modeled after the lodgings of displaced, migrating Plains Indians, here in the Latino heart of the Inland Empire—what better symbol of America's melting pot could there be? *Immigrants*—to quote Alexander Hamilton in the show—*we get the job done.*

We all came here from somewhere. We all rode the same roads to get here. And where we're going, there will always have been others, who did, or didn't, look like us.

We hadn't ventured talking politics or other divisive issues with the people we'd met since Illinois. Perhaps that's what we had gone to escape.

We relaxed and enjoyed the ride—as the art sign along Santa Monica Boulevard urged us on our last stretch toward the Pacific. "UR OK" was a healthy reminder after so many miles.

We arrived, pacified, at the End of the Trail on the Santa Monica Pier, fifteen days after we'd left home. Just one bit of advice: Two weeks wasn't nearly long enough for the drive.

Still, we worried, at times, about the near-term future of our nation. We'd been able to escape that question for a while. But then the roller coaster of our hopes and disappointments grew more drastic than the one we'd passed at Six Flags over Mid-America way back in St. Louis.

What *had* we learned about our Dis-united States?

Back to that Woody Guthrie song we started with. Its message seems fairly simple—we are all equally entitled to the rights of this country, inhabiting and benefiting from the land we stand on. Native Americans, however, readily point out that the core of the song is a colonialist message. Guthrie (1912–1955), as an Anglo resident of Oklahoma growing up among Indian culture, who later said he felt he had something of "a Jewish soul," wasn't unaware of the contradiction.

On our return trip to Tulsa we visited three museums in Guthrie's home state. At the elegant Philbrook, we attended a multimedia performance presenting a range of American songs in the context of American artworks that included two famous larger-than-life portraits of George Washington, along with Benjamin West's enormous 1772 landscape depicting William Penn's treaty with the Indians.

The exhibition aimed to explore American identity through a diverse roster of artists across the centuries. It assembled a stunning array of beautiful and thought-provoking works. Which of these might be seen as culturally inaccurate relics, and which might bring inequities into glaring light? This question, it seemed, was the point of numerous juxtapositions—and here in the heartland we were prompted to ask it of ourselves.

We also spent time in places devoted to the music of visionary folk singers Bob Dylan and Woody Guthrie. In the archives housed at the Woody Guthrie Center, scholar Will Kaufman in 2014 discovered a tranche of writings, letters and song lyrics by Guthrie decrying the racist housing policies of his landlord in Brooklyn, New York, back in the 1950s. That landlord? Fred C. Trump, founder of the family real estate organization.

Guthrie, we learned, originally titled his best-known song "God Blessed America," as visitors can see in his handwritten lyrics on display. Guthrie meant it as a retort to Kate Smith's hit that was sweeping the country in the late 1930s, "God Bless America." While capturing his love of our landscape, he wanted to point out that a lot of Americans weren't feeling too blessed at all.

In 1944, during Word War II, Guthrie revised his song to its now-familiar lyrics and title. It became a hit first in Canada, with localized lyrics, in the mid-1950s and eventually gained traction with many fans, for various causes, from the Sixties onward.

Since then its words have been modified to suit a range of countries, regions, languages, and ethnic groups. Your land and my land may not be the same, but it *was* made for us all, and we have to figure out how to deal with that—sometimes by making peace, sometimes by effecting change.

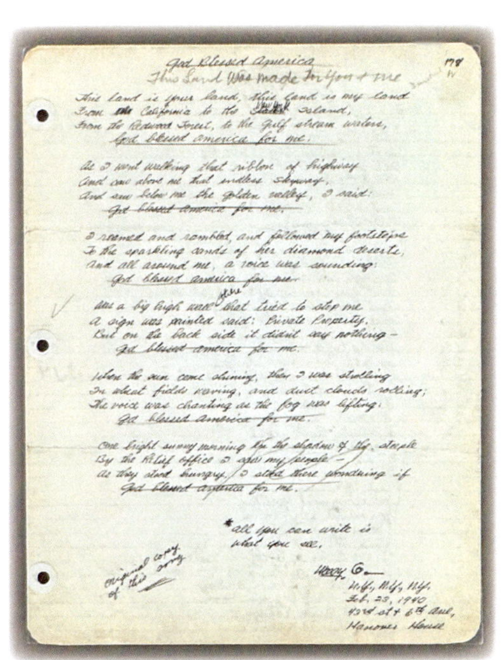

LYRICS ON THE LAND On display under glass at the Woody Guthrie Center in Tulsa, Oklahoma, is a first-draft facsimile of the songwriter's "This Land Is Your Land" from Feb. 23, 1940.

To see and understand not just our world, but ourselves: This is not only why we travel, but why we reflect on the journey, and why we record it for posterity. Why we revisit and revise it. Why we tell our children.

For many of us, the season of political turmoil has been difficult. Sometimes you have to head out on the road and get away.

We have a moral obligation to heal, to be strong, and to get clear-eyed. To vote. To debate. To know our neighbors, and love them as ourselves, regardless of their origins or ideologies.

Looking back at where we've been, at the literal and figurative landscape, helps us chart a better road forward. UR OK, as that sign reminds us.

Keep on, and keep the faith. We'll be fine. ☞

AMERICAN ARTISTS, AMERICAN SONGS was the title of a Nov. 10, 2024 program of "Music on Exhibit" at Tulsa's Philbrook Musem of Art that paired live performances of a song to each of several familiar masterpieces, from Reginald Marsh's "End of the 14th Street Crosstown Line" (1936) projected behind a chamber trio playing a lively Leonard Bernstein piece; or Robinson and Meeropol's vocal number "The House I Live In" sung beneath the James Brantley (left) and Charles Willson Peale (right) paintings projected in the slide.

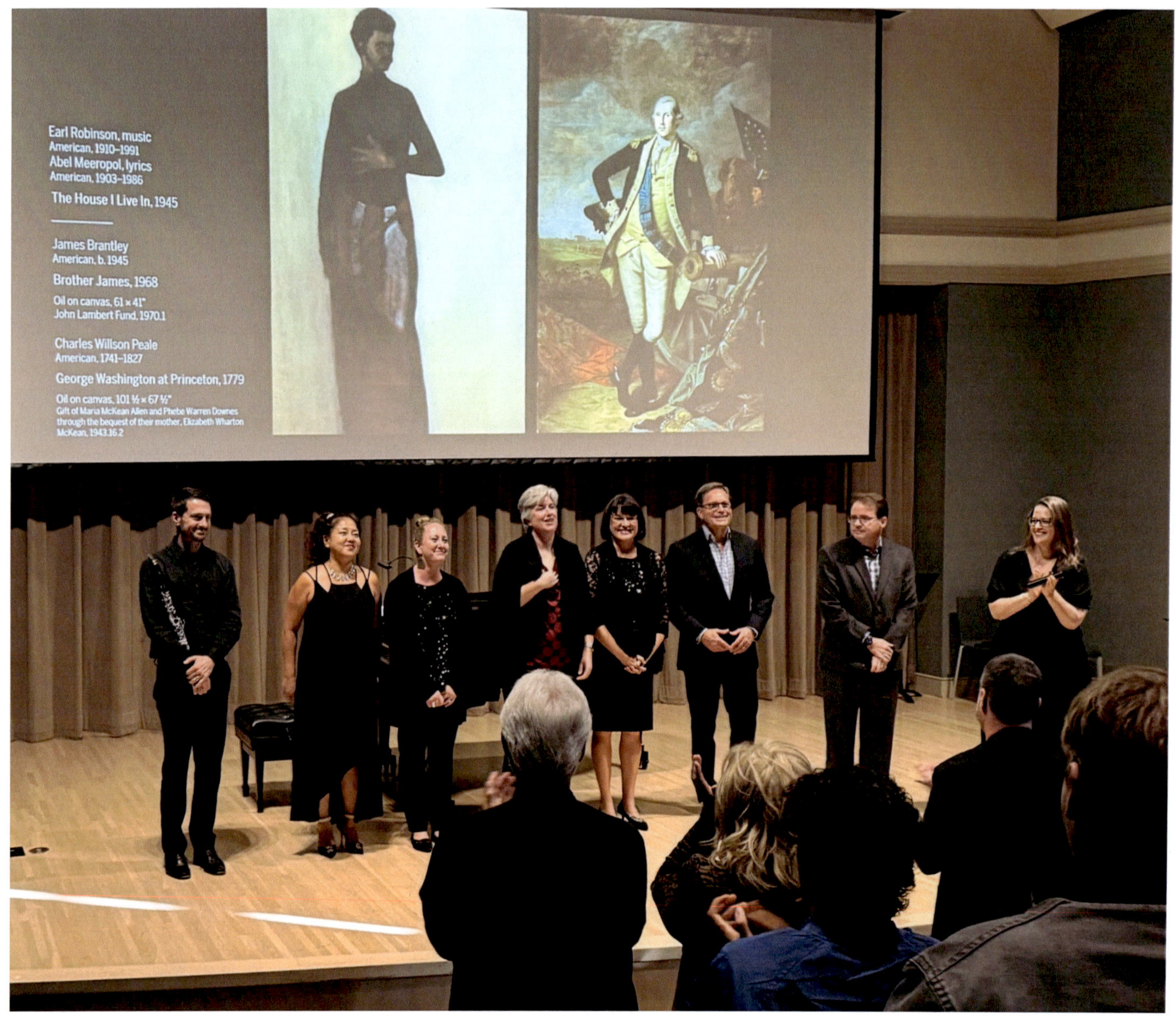

KANSAS PLATES make up an imaginative wall of stars and stripes (right) in Baxter Springs.

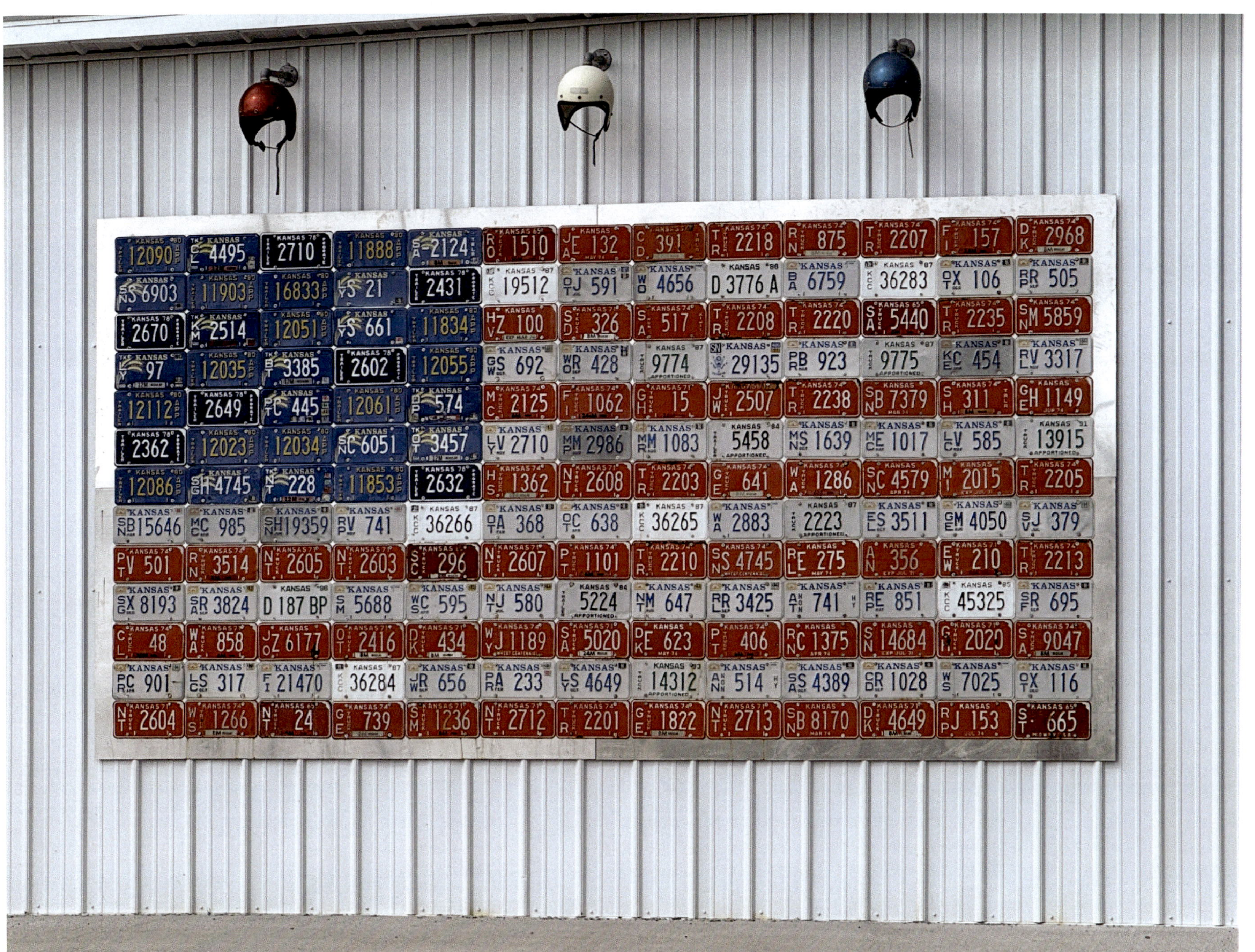

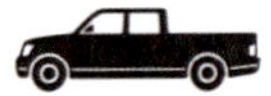

And whither then? I cannot say

BARBARA BRANNON

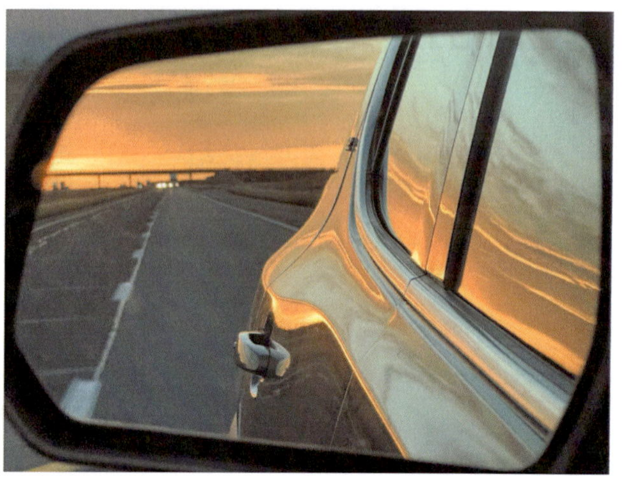

WHEN I GET READY TO TRAVEL, I read up for two reasons: to know something of the history and past culture of the ground I'm about to cover, and to know what resources I need to take along with me. I'm glad to have been reading about Route 66 for decades, since an astonishing body of material has accumulated on the topic for a century and more.

In 2023, the **U.S. National Parks Service Department of the Interior produced the first extended bibliography** on the Mother Road. Even prior to the onslaught of new nonfiction, fiction, and guides churned out just in time for the 2026 Centennial, editors David King Dunaway and Stephen Mandrgoc note "this bibliography *cannot* be considered comprehensive."

But whether you're an academic researcher, a novelist, a writer of guidebooks, or just a casual fan, start here. The pdf is free and worth downloading—all 139 pages of it. https://go.nps.gov/rt66

Beyond this compendium, Kay and I followed an instinctual plan as we undertook this writing and the travel that informed it. Most important, on the approach northward to Chicago we listened (again after many years) to the 2011 Penguin Audio edition of John Steinbeck's *Travels with Charley in Search of America* (1962).

Many Mother Road wanderers have opted, as their road reading, for Steinbeck's 1939 Pulitzer Prize-winning novel **The Grapes of Wrath,** which is credited with first calling Route 66 "the mother road." But we weren't in the mood for the Joads, nor were we keen to revisit Jack Kerouac's 1957 beat novel **On the Road,** which I'd taken along on my first acquaintance with Route 66, in 2023.

Route 66 doesn't lack for audio guides and apps, in English and other languages. AAA, TripAdvisor, and the GuideAlong Gypsy Guides come up at the top of our web searches. But as we weren't seeking turn-by-turn guidance, we found the informative and authentic personality interviews on **Anthony Arno's Route 66 Podcast** to be delightful; on long stretches, the detailed Q&A format didn't bother us a bit.

We enjoyed Rick Antonson's memoir **Route 66** *Still Kicks: Driving America's Main Street* (2013) on Audible as well. Episode 1 begins just where the series ought to: Arno's interview with Michael Wallis.

We tried a few Route-related contemporary novels, but none, to our taste, stood out.

Our essential hard-copy reads:

Michael Wallis, *Route 66: The Mother Road* (New York: St. Martin's, 1990, 256 pages, with color photographs throughout). Having realized I'd left my 2008 paperback at home, I breezed into a secondhand bookshop in Springfield, Illinois, and walked out with a first edition hardcover for ten bucks. A 100th Anniversary edition is due out in May 2026.

Quinta Scott and Susan Croce Kelly, *Route 66: The Highway and Its People* (Norman: University of Oklahoma Press, 1988, 224 pages, with dozens of Scott's excellent black-and-white photos and a very useful index). This research duo contributed greatly to the professional documentation of Route 66 as a historical phenomenon. Their book is still available in the 1990 paperback reprint, but I liked having my hardcover copy on the road with me—even though, as its creators correctly note in the preface, "The history of the road…was a story best learned from the people who knew Route 66 'personally,' and not from books."

Susan Croce Kelly, *Father of Route 66: The Story of Cy Avery* (Norman: University of Oklahoma Press 288 pages, with historical photographs). You can't grasp the significance of the Mother Road without the inspiration of its father, and Kelly's academic but readable biography is essential backstory.

We pre-ordered (shades of fifth-grade social studies projects) or picked up state visitor guides, and were very grateful for their up-to-date location and hours info. We'd purchased a rugged, super-sized plastic accordion folder that happily came with eight subdivisions. It became fuller state by state with our accretion of folding maps, information sheets, postcards, and flat memorabilia.

Jerry McClanahan, *EZ6 Guide for Travelers,* 5th edition (National Historic Route 66 Federation, 2023, spiral bound in state order). If I could live my art life over again, it might well be to draw the kind of building sketches and maps that McJerry has created over the years but craft this essential guidebook with better fonts and less underlining of type. Still, it's a splendidly useful volume, especially if you affix some state-by-state plastic tabs.

Mark Watson, *Route 66 Travel Guide: 202 Amazing Places,* Chicago to Los Angeles Westbound Edition, 2021, paperback, 280 pages. This quirky travel guide is useful for a couple of high-tech reasons: it provides multiple ways to find a particular site (street address, GPS coordinates, and a scannable QR code for each place, that links to your device's navigation)—plus a number-keyed physical map for each state. If the designer were as hip to the usefulness of full page numbers as he is to the trip, you'd quickly be able to locate the QR code for his curated Spotify playlist on page 19, too. As the flip side of McClanahan's linear approach, this guide is worth taking along.

If you're on a bike and not easily able to pull off and scan every code you'd need, consider the **Route 66 Navigation app,** downloadable from Europe-based Touch Media: www.route66navigation.com. We're sign-by-signers rather than turn-by-turners, but the few times we really needed to find a pin from our MapQuest pre-departure estimates, we used this one with success. The array of other options is daunting, and now, AI-assisted as well.

State Route 66 passport booklets, pre-ordered from each state. We loved having these…though our arrival time during open hours of attractions and landmarks proved too iffy for us to collect many stamps. We'll keep adding on future journeys, perhaps far into the future.

Alain de Botton, ***The Art of Travel: A Philosophical Guide to Fulfilling Journeys*** (London, UK: The School of Life, 2018), 132 pages, paperback. This pocket-sized, accessible, London-designed book of travel philosophy provides numerous thought exercises, and a bit of marginal space and extra pages in which to record them.

The section on "How to Come Home" provides this insight to ponder: "Receptivity or openness might be the chief characteristic of the traveler's mindset. As travelers, we approach new places with curiosity. We don't assume we know everything.… We are alive to the layers of a country's history beneath the present" (102).

Rally for the Ribbon Road

Over those Oklahoma hills
Came a newfangled kind of thrill:
A gas-powered transport mode
Folks started calling—"auto-mo-bile."

For buggy lanes the auto wasn't made—
Cars required new surfaces be laid:
Concrete or macadam, brick or plank,
The price to pave the highway must be paid.

Bean counters for the county checked stockpiles,
Fell short by half, in half a dozen trials . . .
When suddenly one pencil-pusher cried:
Divide the lane by half, double the miles!

And so, with a solution engineered,
The bureaucrats were happy, drivers cheered:
Fifteen miles of road, just nine feet wide—
And so the curb was set, the way was cleared.

Sidewalk highway, ribbon road—
Half the cost and twice the miles;
More than eleven decades old,
Half the width, and twice the smiles.
Patch its blacktop if you must,
Or let it crumble into dust,
Fix it for posterity
Or let it be, just wait and see:

But do not ruin the Ribbon Road.
Do not ruin our Ribbon Road.

Rally for our Ribbon Road—
Help us preserve our Ribbon Road.

B.A.B., July 2024

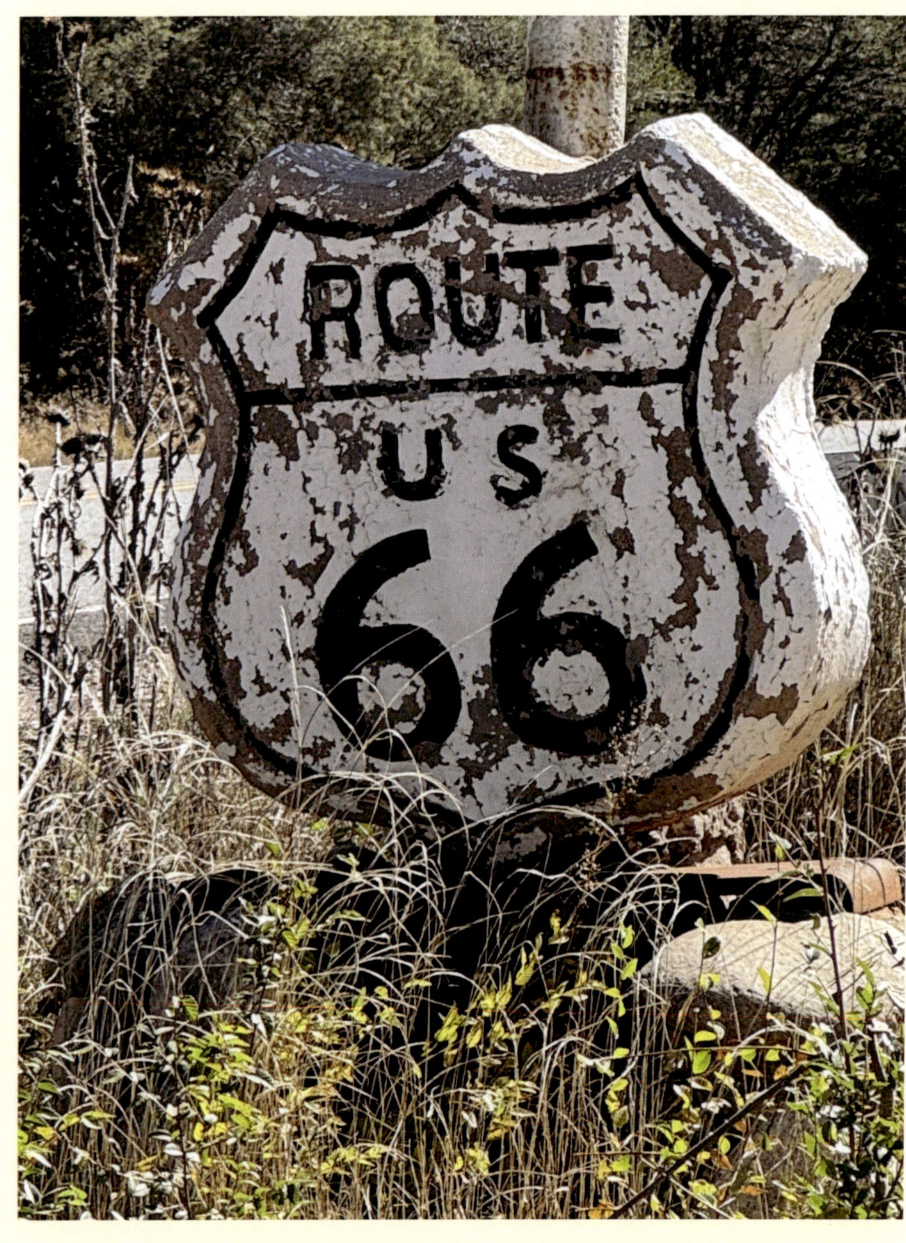

ROUTE RELIC Along the pre-1937 Santa Fe alignment in Glorieta, New Mexico, a giant concrete shield bears the signs of time. For some, the Route 66 experience might seem like a cross-country scavenger hunt for the magic double digits mounted on official highway signposts, painted on walls, stenciled on asphalt, emblazoned on caps and T-shirts.

For us, it was a search for the stories they recall, the people who placed them there, the linked legacy that makes us a nation.

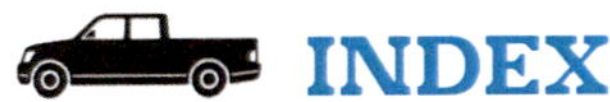 INDEX

9 781935 619659